BURNT OUT

BURNT OUT

The exhausted person's six-step guide to thriving in a fast-paced world

Selina Barker

aster

To all the exhausted and burnt out people out there.
It's time for you to thrive.

First published in Great Britain in 2021 by Aster,
an imprint of
Octopus Publishing Group Ltd
Carmelite House
50 Victoria Embankment
London EC4Y 0DZ
www.octopusbooks.co.uk

An Hachette UK Company
www.hachette.co.uk

Text copyright © Selina Barker 2021
Design and layout copyright © Octopus Publishing Group 2021
Illustrations copyright © Kemal Sanli 2021

Distributed in the US by Hachette Book Group
1290 Avenue of the Americas
4th and 5th floors
New York, NY 10104

Distributed in Canada by Canadian Manda Group
664 Annette St.
Toronto, Ontario, Canada M6S 2C8

ISBN 978 1 78325 400 2

A CIP catalogue record for this book is available from the British Library.

Printed and bound in China

10 9 8 7 6 5 4 3 2 1

Consultant Publisher: Kate Adams
Senior Managing Editor: Sybella Stephens
Copy Editor: Muna Reyal
Art Director: Yasia Williams-Leedham
Designer: Lizzie Ballantyne
Illustrator: Kemal Sanli
Senior Production Manager: Katherine Hockley

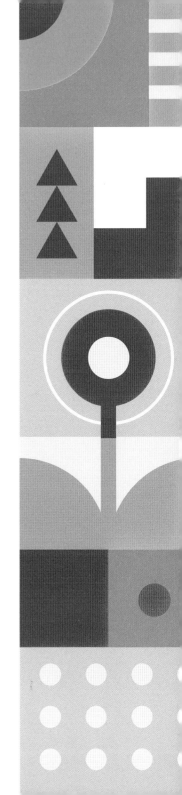

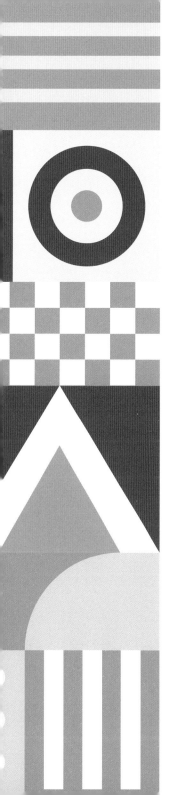

Contents

Introduction

People everywhere are burning out.

From CEOs to nurses, to doctors, teachers, entrepreneurs, journalists, social workers, academics, creatives... even yoga teachers are burning out.

Technology was supposed to make life easier, to free us up, take things *off* our plates, but instead we are feeling more exhausted, more under pressure and more stressed out than ever before. Billions of people all over the world are lying awake at night wired from exhaustion, fearful of the looming to-do list that awaits them in the morning and wondering how the hell they are going to keep this up before they lose the plot altogether.

And not so long ago I was one of those people.

My whole life ran on adrenaline. From the moment I woke up to the moment I went to sleep I was on the go. Busy, busy, busy. Stuck in a constant race against time. Deadlines always looming, work piling up, everything feeling urgent.

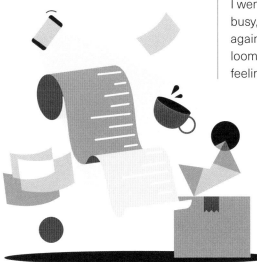

I thought that if I loved my work, then I'd be immune to burnout, but, if anything, I think it made me worse. And it wasn't just work. It was social commitments, family commitments, house admin, appointments to book, shopping to do, laundry to put on, things to buy, emails to answer... the lists were endless. There was never time to pause. The moment something was ticked off the list I moved onto the next.

It all felt too much. I was exhausted. Burnt out on living life. I couldn't see a way for it to stop.

And so, I kept running as fast as I could, afraid that if I did take my foot off the gas, even for a second, my to-do list would catch up with me and beat me mercilessly into the ground.

SURROUNDED BY BURNOUT

I wasn't alone. Everyone around me seemed to be feeling the same.

Then one day, I looked around at my friends and realized that we *all* seemed to be in varying degrees of burnout. Some were suffering the big burnout that has you signed off work for months, others had been hit by yet another mini burnout (that would be me) and some had been living on the brink of burnout for *years*. Finally, I'd had enough of it.

I was done with seeing smart, ambitious, caring people burning out just from trying to live their lives, do their work and look after the people they loved.

I was done with the treadmill, the daily grind and this stupid approach to working, which seemed to suggest that only if you were whipped up into an urgent frenzy would you get all the things done and get to where you wanted to go.

Frankly, I was done with feeling tired and exhausted for what felt like 98 per cent of my life. And while the general mood was 'this is just how modern life is. There's nothing you can do about it', I wasn't having it. Not anymore.

HERE WE GO AGAIN

I'd been here before. Fifteen years ago, as I had stepped into the world of full-time employment, I looked around at the 9–5 existence, the boss, the plastic desk I had to sit at every day and said, 'No way, this is not for me. I don't want to spend the best part of my life sitting in an office all day long, being told what to do and when to do it.'

And I had been met with the same response: 'Yeah, well, no one likes this, but this is just how it is.'

But I wasn't having it then, either.

I knew there were people who were doing it differently. People who were finding a way of making money doing things that they loved, living in a way that gave them the freedom and fulfilment they wanted in life.

I decided that I was going to find those people, learn from them and create my own career doing something that I loved. Then I'd come back and show anyone else that wanted to escape a 9–5 office-based existence how they could do the same.

It worked out pretty well; ten years later I had a career that I *loved as* a life design and career-change coach, that gave me the freedom, creativity, fun, enjoyment, money and fulfilment that I'd once been told was an impossible pipe dream.

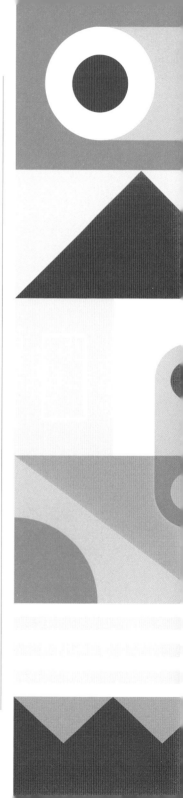

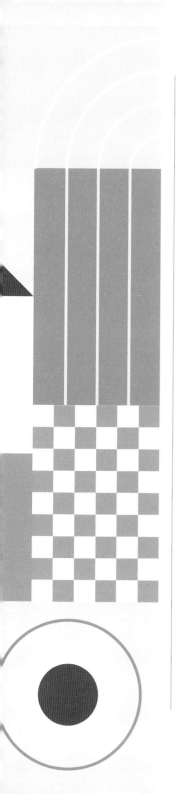

FINDING MY MISSION

So I decided I would do the same again. I would prove that being able to thrive in this fast-paced digital world of ours isn't just a pipe dream – it's what we're here to do.

I knew that life didn't *have* to be this way. That work doesn't *have* to be so stressful that it makes us ill. And that ending every day feeling completely and utterly drained, exhausted and brain frazzled is *not* how it *has* to be.

Over the next few years I dedicated myself to studying, learning and understanding why so many of us seem to be burning out. And, above all, how to break free from the burnout cycle and start to thrive, no matter how hectic the world around us is.

My ultimate goal was to create a practical guide to thriving in a fast-paced modern world for the burnt out, bone tired and brain frazzled. A tool kit to help each of us learn what ingredients and life tools we need in order to thrive, and how to weave those ingredients into our day-to-day lives, no matter how busy life gets. And so here it is: the exhausted person's guide to thriving in a fast-paced world.

Writing this book changed my life. Now I hope it will help you, too.

How to use this book

If you are burnt out right now, or feel that you are rapidly heading that way, then before you go any further, head straight to Burnout SOS (see pages 13–21). Your rest and recovery needs to be your number one priority right now – you do not need to be filling your exhausted head with any other information at this moment.

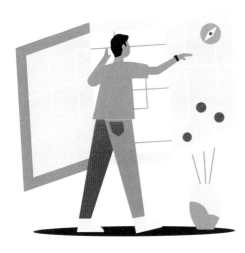

However, if you're feeling ready for change and ready to break free from burnout, then head straight to Part 1 where the journey begins.

As with every transformative journey, it begins by looking inwards. In Part 1 you'll be exploring what inner drivers, fears, stories and limiting beliefs have been causing you to burnout, and I'll be giving you some essential tools to use throughout the journey.

In Part 2 you'll get a crash course on how to reclaim your energy and what you need to be doing day-to-day to keep your physical, emotional and mental energy banks topped up and flowing.

In Part 3 you'll be taking all that you've learnt in Part 2 and using it to design your life so that you can thrive. We'll be looking in particular at how to design your working day.

And if you know that some bigger things in your life need to change – perhaps your job, your career, how you work or where you live – then we'll be looking at how to make those bigger changes too.

This book isn't just something to read once, but is a guide and a toolkit that you can come back to whenever you need to remind yourself what you need in your life to thrive and be happy.

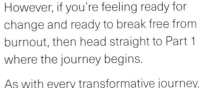

THIS BOOK CAN'T CHANGE YOUR LIFE, BUT...

I promise you that the tools and exercises in this book can completely turn your life around.

Not only will they help you to recover from burnout, but they will show you how to design your life and form new habits and rituals that will have you living with more energy, vitality and power than you ever have before, BUT... you have to *use* it.

Reading this book alone won't bring about change but doing the exercises will. And for that you have to create the space and time to do it.

I know if you're run off your feet or feeling totally defeated by life at the moment then finding time can seem hard, but you *can* do it and you *need* to do it.

Don't wait for the time to magically appear – it won't. Don't wait until you *feel* like doing it. As much as you might think you want to thrive and feel energized, trust me there will be a big part of you that will want to remain stuck and will resist doing this work. So, you have to *commit* to doing it.

Choose when and at what time you want to commit to working through this book, then schedule it into your calendar or diary and put a reminder on your phone if need be.

And if, after booking in dates in your calendar, you *still* don't do it, ask someone that loves you to be your accountability buddy. Someone you can check in with once a week to share how you're getting on, celebrate each step you take forward and encourage you to get back on track when you inevitably fall off (and it will happen – it happens to all of us, no matter how enthusiastic we are when we get started).

Burnout SOS

If you're currently in full-blown burnout or feeling on the brink of burnout, before we move on we need to make your rest and recovery the *only* focus right now. The rest of this book can wait until after you've had some proper R&R and not a moment before.

Help!

I am in full-blown burnout

People burnout in different ways.

Some people feel so physically exhausted that they can barely get out of bed. Others feel desperately tired but are so jacked up on adrenaline, they can't get to sleep when they try and wrestle with insomnia and restless nights. Others feel emotionally raw and exhausted and find themselves bursting into tears at the smallest things.

Some lose all compassion and stop caring about a career they once used to love. Others become cynical and start doubting what they once believed in. Some get physically ill or find themselves having accidents and making silly mistakes they wouldn't normally make, like locking themselves out of their home or getting on the wrong train.

Some feel a total loss in confidence and no longer feel they can do a job that they were once good at. Others feel as if a fuse has gone in their brain – they are slow, foggy, struggle to focus, are suddenly very forgetful and find that even the smallest decision feels impossible to make.

While burn-out symptoms can be different from one person to the next, everyone shares one thing in common: total and utter exhaustion.

The symptoms of burnout:

- Physical exhaustion
- Trouble sleeping
- Loss of compassion
- Stopped caring about your job
- Physical illness
- Making mistakes you wouldn't usually make
- Loss of confidence
- Fogginess
- Loss of focus
- Doubting your abilities
- Cynicism
- Procrastination
- Pessimism
- Crying
- Inability to concentrate
- Feeling unable to cope

TIME TO TAKE ACTION

These are all signs that your body has had enough. It wants you to stop and you need to listen. You need to treat this as if you have really bad flu – your priority now needs to be rest.

Cancel your plans, turn off your phone. Talk to someone that loves you and let them know how you're feeling.

If you're feeling in any way scared about your mental health, do not hesitate to speak to a professional. You need to feel held and supported right now.

And breathe.

You're going to be OK.

YOUR PRIORITY NOW NEEDS TO BE:

- Sleep
- Rest
- More sleep
- Relaxation (hot bath or shower)
- Comfy clothes
- Calming your nervous system (tips on how to do that can be found on page 96)
- Nourishing your body (and when I say nourishing, I absolutely think that this can include ice cream and biscuits, but hold off the booze)
- Feeling your feelings (find a tool to help you do that on page 137)
- Letting yourself be supported by others

Don't try to figure stuff out. Don't try planning your future. This is not the time to be making big life decisions.

And, quite frankly, your brain probably doesn't have the juice left in it to think beyond what you're going to have for dinner. It might not even be able to handle that.

Let your mind and body REST.

Now, if you've had a mini burnout, you might find that a weekend or a week is enough to help you recover, particularly if you really take the rest and recovery seriously. But a big burnout takes longer to recover from and you might need to take a proper break from work. I interviewed a lot of people who had taken a few months off from work to recover from burnout – they needed it. See your doctor about getting signed off work and, if you work for a company, speak to your boss or HR.

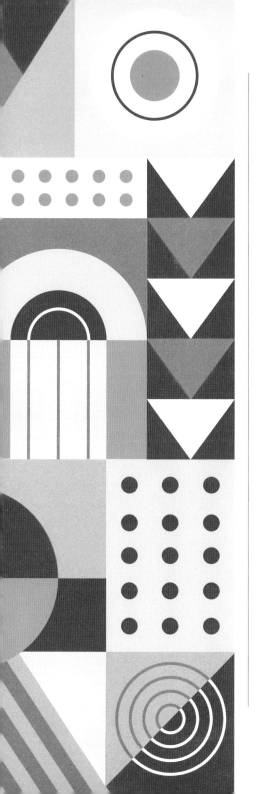

DESIGN YOUR 'RECOVERY FROM BURNOUT' DAYS

When you're recovering from burnout, taking care of yourself, resting and doing things that help lift your spirits is your number one and *only* job.

Do not turn this time out into an opportunity to get things done around the house, and don't you *dare* use it to catch up on your to-do list.

Your full focus needs to be on spending your time doing things that will really nourish you and help you to get your energy back up.

Activities to help you to rest, nourish yourself and lift your spirits:

- Getting out in nature
- Walking
- Gentle exercise
- Swimming
- Meditation
- Reading in bed
- Cooking
- Eating nourishing food
- Gardening
- Talking to people
- Getting creative
- Making things
- Watching films that make you laugh
- Journalling
- Staring out of the window and doing nothing
- Listening to your favourite music
- Playing a game

TAKING TIME OUT

- Create a light structure to your day. Waking up and having nothing planned in your day could leave you feeling a bit lost and anxious, but scheduling too many things could leave you feeling overwhelmed. So, have a go at planning just one or two simple things for the day – maybe one thing in the morning and one thing after lunch, and see how you go.
- Switch off fully from work. FULLY. No chatting to work friends to find out what's going on, no checking emails once a day in case anything is important. You won't be able to recover if you are still plugged into work. If you need help switching off (which a *lot* of us do), head to page 193 for some tips on how to do that.
- Switch off the notifications on your phone and, if you find yourself on social media a lot, I recommend removing the apps from your phone too for now (you can put them back later).
- Talk to loving and supportive people.
- Eat lots of nourishing food.
- Drink plenty of water.
- Sleep

When you feel ready and your mind doesn't feel overwhelmed at the idea of taking on new information, you can head on into the next section of this book and we'll get you started on reclaiming back your energy and your life.

But only when you really do feel ready.

Don't try to rush your recovery.

Help!

I can feel a burnout coming on

If you are used to having mini burnouts, you'll know what it's like when it starts to come on:

- Everything starts to feel urgent, the pressure is building and time feels horribly scarce.

- You start trying to squeeze work into the times you know you should be resting. You start dropping the self-care practices you *know* are so important. Suddenly anything other than work feels like a luxury. *There just isn't the time.*

- You are tired and wired. You know you're running on empty, but you don't feel you have any other option than to carry on, so you override your body's very clear message that you need to rest and recharge, and push yourself on with coffee, sugar, alcohol or sheer determination.

When this starts to happen, hard though it is to slam on the brakes, that is exactly what you need to do. You need to make rest and recharge an immediate priority.

If you need any convincing, then just remind yourself that if you don't and you fully burnout, you will be out of action for days if not weeks, so if you catch it now, you'll save yourself a lot of time and a lot of tears.

You need to book in some proper rest and recovery time ASAP. Decide right this moment when you can do that and what you will do to help calm your nervous system, make rest a priority and recharge your batteries.

What doesn't work, is to grab a bottle of wine on the way home, flop on the sofa to watch TV and scroll mindlessly through your phone and then crawl into bed way past bedtime. It might *feel* like it's what you want to do, but it is definitely not what your body or brain need you to do.

So, what are the early warning signs that you're slipping into overdrive and starting to burn yourself out? What really helps you to relax, rest and recharge your batteries when you're starting to feel burnt out? And what *doesn't* work so well?

For as long as you are still feeling exhausted and stressed, keep prioritising rest and recovery until you start to feel your energy coming back, your mind feels clearer and your heart happier.

Why are we burning out?

Burnout is a level of mental, emotional and physical exhaustion that a nice cup of tea and a hot bath just won't cure. It's the feeling that you simply can't cope any more – that you haven't got what it takes – and you're not sure you can go on.

Burnout has become such a global occurrence that in May 2019 the WHO classified it as a medical condition: 'an occupational phenomenon resulting from chronic workplace stress that has not been successfully managed.' In Japan they even have a word that means death from burnout: 'Karoshi'.

So, what is going on? What has happened to get us working at such a pace and under so much pressure that it's driving so many of us into burnout? And, most importantly, what can we do about it?

A modern-day problem?

For the best part of six months I dived into the topic of burnout to try to answer these questions. I read every book, article and study I could find. I interviewed people who had recovered from burnout, people who were in the middle of burnout and people who felt it wasn't far off.

I wanted to try and get to the heart of the problem: why were so many of us burning out?

Is it modern life? Toxic work cultures? Crappy bosses? Poor leadership? The Patriarchy? Systemic racism?

A post-industrialist work culture that has taught us to think we can operate like machines? Is it our new age of digital technology that has seduced us into staying switched on 24/7?

Or is it that open-plan offices that create an environment of non-stop interruptions that is literally driving us to distraction?

A modern-day addiction to busyness? A totally misguided belief that being stressed is a sign that you're working really hard and fast?

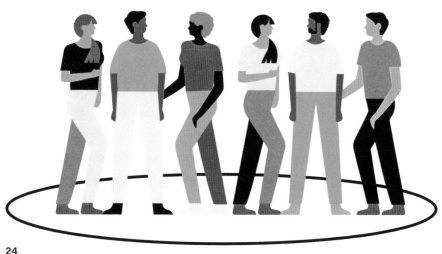

An age-old patriarchal obsession with progress and productivity?

A capitalist society that has us all chasing after the extrinsic goals of money, status, popularity, image, keeping us hooked on outside achievement and validation from others because we think that will lead to happiness and success (but it never does)?

A deep-rooted belief that a good and caring person, particularly a good woman, is someone that lives to serve the needs of others and therefore shouldn't be so selfish or greedy as to ask that their needs should be fulfilled? Are we hard-wired to strive and struggle, even when we do have the opportunity to thrive? Or is it just that we're all really, really bad at looking after ourselves and putting ourselves first?

Well, in a nutshell, YES. It's all of the above. And a whole lot more.

It's also an unjust, unequal and unfair world that is addicted to more, more, more, faster, faster, faster and it is jam-packed with toxic bosses and toxic work cultures.

TAKING CONTROL

The fact is that the modern world we live in today is not designed for most of us to thrive.

But does that mean we *can't* thrive?

Hell no.

What it means is that we have to take things into our own hands.

It is time to take a radical new approach, not only to the way we live and work, but to the way we take care of ourselves. One that helps us to remain calm, grounded and energized, no matter how hectic life gets. And that is what this book is all about.

I'm going to show you the tools that you need to rise up and reclaim your energy and your life.

- I'm going to show you how to go from feeling utterly exhausted and brain frazzled to feeling calmer, more energized and more in control of your life than ever before.
- I'm going to show you how to set yourself free from your never-ending to-do lists, cure your addiction to busyness (yes, it is an addiction) and discover simple and effective ways to stop yourself from spinning out on stressful days.
- And I'm going to show you how to become so energized, calm and focused at work that everyone will be asking you what your secret is.
- And, most important of all, I'm going to make it as easy as possible for you to do, guiding you to the parts of the book that will help you most right now to get your energy back and start designing a life that you can thrive in.

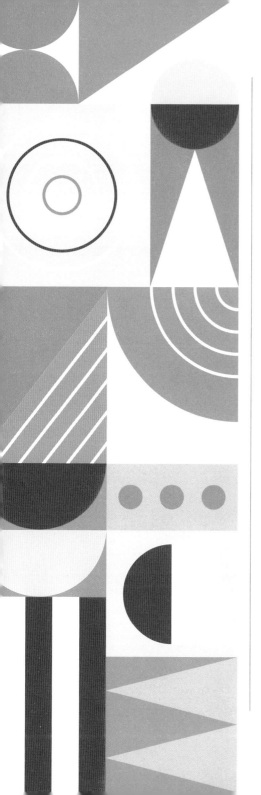

LEARNING HOW TO THRIVE

Working out how to thrive in a fast-paced modern world isn't complicated. All the things you will need to do in order to feel energized, calm and grounded on a day-to-day basis are things you already know how to do. What is going to be hard is actually *doing* those things. Even though right now you may say that yes, of course, you want to thrive in life, of course you want to feel energized, calm and grounded day after day – trust me,

you

will

resist

it.

Almost all of us resist making our happiness and well-being a top priority in life, particularly those of us with a tendency to stress and burnout. In fact, we can be some of the worst at looking after ourselves, which is in part how we got ourselves into this burnt-out mess in the first place.

Now, I know there might have been big, outside factors that also played a critical role in your burnout. And I'm not for a second underplaying the exhaustion and psychological pain that can come from doing traumatic frontline work, having a toxic boss or from discrimination in the workplace and society – we will get onto that. But right at the heart of this burnout epidemic is a universal reluctance to look after ourselves properly so that we can thrive in life – either because we don't know how to do it or because we don't allow ourselves the possibility to do it.

For most of us it's a mixture of both.

Because almost every person I have ever met has been brought up to believe that their self-care and their needs are not a priority.

That if you're a good, responsible and caring person, you will put your needs to one side and dedicate yourself to attending to the needs of others, particularly if you're a woman or a care giver. And if you're a mother, then you shouldn't have needs at all, the very role of raising children and looking after your family should be fulfilment enough.

If your parents, grandparents or ancestors experienced famine, poverty, enslavement, war or trauma you may carry strong inner beliefs that you simply can't rest and relax, that it's not *safe* to do that. That you must always strive, struggle and fight to survive. I have often found clients experience a strong sense of guilt at the idea that they could thrive and be happy if their families or ancestors never had that opportunity. As if by making their own self-care a priority, they are somehow abandoning and betraying those that came before them.

On the surface, while learning to look after yourself and thriving can seem like a no-brainer (we all want that, right?), there are powerful forces at play beneath the surface that will have you resisting it, no matter how much you might think you want it.

The biggest challenge of all on this journey will be overcoming your resistance to making your well-being and happiness a priority in your life.

This journey has to begin with you making a commitment. A commitment to change, a commitment to taking action and, above all, a commitment to focus on you.

The six steps to take you from burnout to thriving

STEP 1

Commit to making your happiness and wellbeing a top priority in your life.

STEP 2

Get to know your inner Shitty Committee and how it is driving you to burn out.

STEP 3

Tune into your inner Wise Cheerleader and turn up the volume.

STEP 4

Learn how to become a master at managing your own energy.

STEP 5

Design your life so that you can thrive.

STEP 6

Bring about big change when the people or environments around you are causing you to burn out.

PART 1

TAKE A LOOK INSIDE OF YOU

To begin your journey of reclaiming your energy and learning how to thrive, first we need to understand what has been going on under the surface causing you to burn out in the first place.

Every transformation in life starts from within. Whether you want to move into a different career, transform your love life or learn how to thrive – any change is always going to be an inside-out job.

While there are likely to be some significant outside factors that have been contributing to your burnout: a heavy workload; a demanding boss; a baby who won't sleep; difficult clients; long work hours; a toxic work culture; a job that is making you miserable – all things that we will be addressing later on in the book – we first have to shine a light on what is going on inside that could be driving you to the point of utter exhaustion and burnout.

And to do that we need to get acquainted with what I like to affectionately call your inner Shitty Committee.

Introducing your Shitty Committee

Your Shitty Committee is the negative, critical, fear-mongering voice in your head that loves nothing more than to point out all the mistakes you're making, all the things you should be worrying about, why something probably won't work, why it's best to just stick to what you know and all the many ways you are simply not good enough.

Your Shitty Committee is the ultimate party pooper. It is also most definitely the reason you burnt yourself out.

Your Shitty Committee is what sends you into overdrive, whip in hand, filling you with warnings about what will happen if you don't meet that deadline, don't get that promotion, don't work hard enough or fast enough. When you're in panic mode, having a melt down or a crisis of confidence or an area of your life where you feel stuck, you can be sure that your Shitty Committee is right by your side, fuelling the fire of doubt and fear within you.

And so, this is where your journey to breaking free from the burn-out cycle needs to begin. We need to get to know your Shitty Committee – what stories it's telling you, what limiting beliefs it is having you live by and, in particular, which of those stories and limiting beliefs are driving you to burn out.

So, let's start by taking a closer look at how you tend to behave when your Shitty Committee is in town and whipping you up into a frenzied state.

What's your burn-out archetype?

Your burn-out archetype is how you tend to behave when your Shitty Committee is in town.

When the pressure is on, suddenly everything feels urgent and you kick into fight-or-flight mode.

Your burn-out archetype is in fact the shadow side of your greatest strengths, jacked up on adrenaline, driven by fear and gone a little loco.

Read through some of the common archetypes on the following pages and you might recognize yourself in more than one. You might even recognize yourself in all of them – I certainly do.

The key point to remember here is that this is not *who* you are, it's just a way you can find yourself behaving when you've gone into overdrive and stress is running the show.

The Over-doer

The over-doer is the shadow side of the naturally resourceful and practical person who, when they are in their full power, takes on the challenges of the day with a positive can-do attitude, ease and enthusiasm.

But when the Shitty Committee is in town and they slip into overdrive, they lose their carefree ease and enthusiasm and turn into a serious over-doer.

You know when you've slipped into over-doer mode because you suddenly start working like a maniac as if your life depends on it. There suddenly seems to be a never-ending, overwhelming amount that needs to be done. And it all feels urgent. You seem to be non-stop. Can't sit still. Can't relax. You suddenly seem to be insanely busy. Your schedule is jam-packed, juggling work, home, family and social commitments. You grind through your to-do list day after day like a machine. There is little joy in it as you don't feel as if you have an option. You'd love to rest, love to do the things you enjoy, but there simply isn't time. Or so you keep telling yourself and others.

Because the truth is even when you do have time to rest and relax and take a break from your to-do list, the chances are, you don't. You are driven by the constant need to be doing. You are addicted to being busy.

You are a product of a culture that rewards hard work, progress and productivity, and dismisses stillness and rest. And so on you go, trapped on the treadmill, feeling that you can never jump off, not realizing that you're the one keeping you on there.

When burnout is coming on, the wheels start to feel like they're coming off.

Despite how fast you seem to be doing everything, it all seems to take twice as long as it normally should, which makes you even more anxious.

'*There's not enough time*' is your panicked mantra.

Everything feels urgent and life feels as if it is spinning out of control and you can't keep up with it.

You start to feel like you are being crushed by your daily responsibilities and the never-ending to-do list.

Work just keeps piling up.

You feel exhausted.

You are prone to making mistakes you wouldn't normally make.

There is nothing worse for you than feeling like you are inefficient or incapable and, to your horror, here you are feeling inefficient and incapable.

When burnout hits, you feel tired to the core.

Physically drained and worn out.

You might get ill after chronic stress weakens your immune system or you simply feel like you can't get out of bed.

You also might find yourself having an accident that forces you to get into bed and rest.

The Over-giver

The over-giver is the shadow side of the naturally loving, caring person who feels deeply for others. They are the person who others turn to for help and they are deeply motivated and fulfilled by being of service and helping those in need.

But when the Shitty Committee is in town and they slip into overdrive, all their self-care and self-love practices go out the window and they become the over-giver, focused on how they can help everyone else and forgetting (often refusing) to let others help them.

You'll know when you've slipped into over-giver mode because you'll find yourself suddenly helping everyone else out while your own work and self-care seem to fall lower and lower down your list of priorities.

You'll find it almost impossible to say no to people, even though you're struggling to keep on top of everything as it is.

You can feel as if you have very little time for yourself because you're focused 24/7 on everyone else's needs instead of your own.

When burnout is coming on, you can feel your cup running dry.

You feel like you've got very little left to give.

You can find yourself feeling more and more depleted by helping others.

You feel spread too thin and can start to feel increasingly guilty about not being able to be there for people in the way you'd like to be and quietly resenting that no one else seems to be noticing that you need help, too.

Normally you love helping or caring for people, but now it's starting to feel like a chore, a burden, an obligation.

When burnout hits, you are emotionally exhausted.

You can either find yourself retreating and making yourself small or making those closest to you feel guilty for not meeting your needs.

You deprive yourself of the things that bring you pleasure and may stop your self-care habits as a form of self-punishment and martyrdom.

You can find yourself feeling empty, negative, resentful, lonely, sad and even depressed.

You might feel as if you don't recognize yourself any more – you used to be so caring and compassionate and now it feels as if you have lost your ability to care. With that can come a big identity crisis, particularly if you are a parent and/or in a caring profession.

Your Shitty Committee can get nasty and you can feel like you're not sure you can carry on.

The Over-thinker

The over-thinker is the shadow side of the naturally smart thinker, problem solver, intellectual or inventor. They have a brilliant mind that is able to come up with solutions and ideas like no one else.

But, when the Shitty Committee is in town and they slip into overdrive, the calm and focus disappears and their thinking becomes obsessive and urgent.

You'll know when you've slipped into over-thinker mode, because your thinking will go into hyper-speed.

Your mind will race and you'll find you can't stop thinking, even when you try. Because if *you* don't figure it out, who will?!

You'll feel like a brain in a jar, living from the neck up, barely aware of the rest of your body or its needs.

You'll struggle to switch off from work at the end of the day and might have problems falling asleep or waking up in the middle of the night worrying about things.

When burnout is coming on, you feel brain-frazzled and fried.

You start to feel foggy, struggle to concentrate or to hold your focus for long and, if you're in a creative job, you might find that your creativity seems to be drying up.

When burnout hits, your brain feels like it has given up.

A fuse has gone and even the simplest decisions can feel totally overwhelming.

You are wired and tired.

Your anxiety can be at an all-time high and panic attacks aren't uncommon.

The Over-achiever

The over-achiever is the shadow side of the bold, visionary, creative, entrepreneur or leader who loves to make things happen. They have strong visions and clear goals and are lit up by the ideas they are bringing to life. They often have multiple exciting, projects on the go at any one time.

But when the Shitty Committee is in town and they slip into overdrive, their energy and enthusiasm is replaced with a dogged grit and determination.

You'll know when you've slipped into over-achiever mode because your projects will stop feeling fun and start feeling like gruelling challenges. All you will think about is work and what you have to do next.

People will be impressed at how much you get done and the speed at which you do it. But it comes at a cost. What people don't realize is that you can't stop and you're miserable. Your drive is literally driving you. Your inner battle is often with perfectionism, imposter syndrome or both. Whether you are driven by a need to make a difference, a need to make great work/art, a need to succeed or a need to make more money, it's like an addiction. Because underneath it all is the deep, driving fear of failure and of ultimately being found out that you're not good enough.

When burnout is coming on, you stop playing and you get serious.

You become like a machine.

You become obsessed with your work and can become irritable and impatient with the people around you.

Your Shitty Committee keeps snapping its whip, driving you on, reminding you of how catastrophic it will be if you fail.

On the inside you start to lose confidence and start to doubt your abilities, while on the outside, you can be defensive and quick to blame others or you retreat, go inwards and shut the rest of the world out.

When burnout hits, you crash hard.

Your body has wisely brought you to your knees.

You can't go on.

Sometimes it is simply that your body can no longer handle the stress and you become mentally or physically ill; sometimes it is triggered by a disappointment with your work – a goal isn't met, a project falls apart or you don't get the job.

Suddenly all the built-up stress kicks in and takes you down.

You retreat from the world feeling like a total failure.

You can't bear to reach out and might feel reluctant to respond when people reach out to you, wanting to help.

WHICH BURNOUT ARCHETYPE ARE YOU?

As I said, you might recognize yourself in a few or *all* of them, so take a moment now to think about how you tend to behave when the pressure is on and you kick into overdrive. Which of these behaviours sound most like you when you're stressed out and heading into burnout?

The over-doer, over-giver, over-thinker and over-achiever aren't *who* you are. They are simply sides of you that come out when you're under pressure and your Shitty Committee is in town, filling you with doubts and fears that throw you into a panic and send you into overdrive. The problem is that if you have a Shitty Committee who is by your side 24/7, then you can find yourself stuck operating from your burn-out archetype from the moment you wake up to the moment you collapse into bed. And when that happens, burnout is inevitable.

So, in order to break free from the burn-out cycle and learn how to thrive, the first thing you need to do is learn how to turn down the volume of your Shitty Committee.

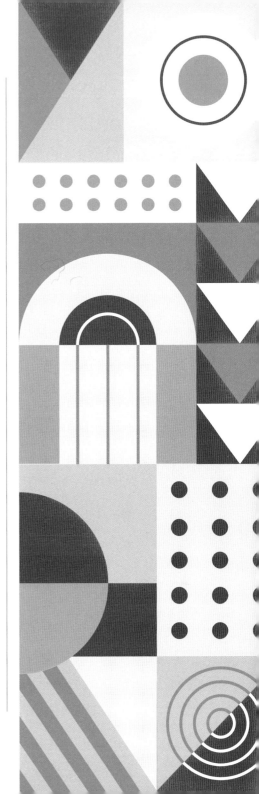

How to handle your Shitty Committee

The reason that the Shitty Committee can have such an influence over us and can be such a powerful force in our lives is because we *believe* the limiting beliefs it is feeding us.

We believe that what it is saying to us is *THE TRUTH*. It's not.

But it feels like it is because the Shitty Committee has been spending years, most of your life in fact, pointing out evidence to back up what it's saying, so it feels as if those beliefs *are* the truth.

In addition to that, you might have noticed that your Shitty Committee often sounds very similar to a certain family member or someone who had a strong influence over you as you were growing up. And so when your inner Shitty Committee and people in your outer world are saying the same thing, it can be easy to believe that what they are all saying is true.

And because we create our reality to align with our beliefs, we then find ourselves unwittingly creating a reality to match what our Shitty Committee is telling us.

If your Shitty Committee tells you you're hopeless with money, constantly reminds you of all the times you've struggled with money, how often you are in overdraft and compares you to friends who always seem to have lots of money then, lo and behold, you'll just keep staying stuck in a space of money scarcity no matter how hard you think you're trying to get out of it.

Because your beliefs shape your reality.

If you think life is a struggle, that being an adult is stressful, that you have to strive to survive, then you are going to create your life and make choices so that you can live out that reality. You will seek out the struggle, the stress and the jobs and situations that prove you and your Shitty Committee right.

So, in order for you to be able to give up the struggling and start to thrive, you need to learn how to handle your Shitty Committee and set yourself free from its limiting beliefs.

TURN UP THE VOLUME ON YOUR SHITTY COMMITTEE

To turn down the volume on your Shitty Committee, first you have to turn its volume UP to hear whatever negative and limiting beliefs it is feeding you, and then find evidence to prove it WRONG.

Think about something that is really important to you at the moment – a positive change you want to make in your life or a dream you really want to make happen.

Write it down:

I REALLY WANT

- To be happy
- To dedicate time everyday to exercise + fitness
- love my job again
- do more consistently

If your mind is drawing a blank (not uncommon when you're burnt out), try some of these:

'I really want to live my life feeling happy and energized.'

'I really want to have a career that I love.'

'I really want to always have an abundance of money and my savings increasing every month.'

Now, unleash that negative, critical Shitty Committee of yours. What does it have to say about this, about you and why your dream won't happen? And don't hold back. Write down all the negative, limiting, critical things your Shitty Committee has to say.

Why does your Shitty Committee say it won't happen?

not good enough
lazy
tired
not organized enough
need to make other goals
need money
no other experience
don't know who I am
don't know my interests
to do
to late
not enough time to figure it out
to busy

I want you to take a moment and recognize how it feels when your Shitty Committee is saying all this stuff to you and *you're believing it.*

It doesn't exactly inspire you to spring into action and start making that dream happen, does it? That is *why* you need to learn how to handle your Shitty Committee. Because without you even realizing it, it could be having a huge impact on your life, burning you out and holding you back.

STEP **2**	**PROVE YOUR SHITTY COMMITTEE WRONG**	For every negative belief that your Shitty Committee is feeding you, you need to find evidence or an argument to prove it wrong. Here are some examples:

The SHITTY COMMITTEE says	Evidence to prove it WRONG
This new business idea of yours is nothing more than a pipedream. You're going to fail and make a fool of yourself.	Every idea starts as a dream – lots of my ideas have started as a pipedream and yet I've made a lot of them happen already, such as that trip I made to South America and my dream of finding a home I could afford to live in on my own. I believed in those pipedreams and I made them happen. If THIS business idea doesn't work out, then I will learn from it, adapt the idea and try again. I'm not afraid of failure and you're not going to put me off giving this my best shot.
If you don't meet that deadline it will be a disaster. It's not professional. They'll realize that you're not good enough. So you better pull an all-nighter to get it done.	If I don't meet that deadline no one is going to die. We might have to move a few meetings around, but better to do that than hand over work that has been finished off in a hurry in the middle of the night when I know I won't be producing my best work. It is more important that this work is at its best than that the deadline be met. Failure would be to not speak up and let them know in advance that I'll need a little more time, and destroy myself trying to meet a deadline that was too tight anyway. I've been working hard on this and they all know that.
It's too late to make a career change. Just be grateful that you even have a job.	There are loads of people who have made successful career changes when they were older than me. And while I'm grateful that I have a job, I'd never forgive myself for settling for this when I know I can do so much more with my life and career.

Now it's your turn – fill in the table overleaf.

If you find yourself stuck and unable to come up with any evidence to prove your Shitty Committee wrong, ask a good supportive friend to help. I bet you they will be able to come up with loads of evidence. It's always a lot easier to handle someone else's Shitty Committee than it is to handle your own. In fact, it can be a lot of fun. So, don't be afraid to ask a friend for help if you need it. They'll enjoy it!

Once you start coming up with evidence to prove your Shitty Committee wrong you'll notice that what it is saying doesn't make you so upset any more, and that is when you know its volume is starting to go down and it is losing its power over you.

That simple act of being able to liberate yourself from your own limiting beliefs is, honestly, life changing.

You can use this simple but powerful tool any time that you feel upset, angry, panicked or stressed out about something. Just ask yourself, 'What is my Shitty Committee saying about this and about *me*?' And then get to work challenging every belief it is feeding you. You'll be amazed at how quickly it can help you to shift your perspective, moving you back into a positive headspace, where you believe in yourself and what you want to achieve.

What my SHITTY COMMITTEE says	Evidence to prove it WRONG

What my SHITTY COMMITTEE says

Evidence to prove it WRONG

CREATE A NEW SET OF EMPOWERING BELIEFS

Once you've proved your Shitty Committee wrong, you can use the evidence to disempower it and create a new set of empowering beliefs to remind you that you *can* make this happen, you *have* got this.

For example, Sade wants this to be the year where she starts her own business.

Her Shitty Committee is afraid she will fail and has been saying that she doesn't have what it takes to make it happen. She points out to her Shitty Committee all the ways that she has worked through challenges before, even when she didn't know what she was doing. She's read loads of inspiring stories of women who have started their own business and said that failure is all part of the journey. Plus, she'd rather try and fail than not try at all. You can learn from failure, but you can't learn from doing nothing.

Her new belief is: 'I am dedicated and committed to bringing this new business idea into the world next year. I can ask for help if and when I need it, be inspired by other women in business and learn the skills I need to make this happen. The only real failure is the failure to try.'

Now it's your turn. Taking a look at the evidence you used to prove your Shitty Committee wrong, how can you turn that into a new empowering belief that really supports you in making this dream of yours happen?

My new empowering belief is:

How would it feel to live by this new belief?

How would believing this make you behave and act differently?

What would you start to do differently that you're not doing now?

Now start beliveing it.

Repeat it to yourself every day and notice how the more you repeat it, the more you start to truly believe it. And the more you start to truly believe it, the more action you'll take in this area of your life, helping it to become a reality.

Because that is the power of belief.

Keep challenging what the Shitty Committee is saying and allow your new beliefs to help you step back into your power as you go on this journey of reclaiming your energy and your life.

Say hello to your inner Wise Cheerleader

OK, there is one more aspect of yourself that I'm keen for you to meet. It's what I like to call your inner Wise Cheerleader. But you can call it your inner Wise One, inner guide, inner Mr Miyagi... whatever works for you to conjure up a wise, supportive voice within you.

It is the *opposite* to your Shitty Committee.

Rather than making you feel bad and giving you a hard time, your inner Wise Cheerleader is totally focused on your happiness and well-being, and will offer guidance, kindness, compassion, LOLs and pep talks whenever you need them.

Your friends probably know this side of you well. They probably get your inner Wise Cheerleader talking to them all the time. It's only you that ends up stuck listening to your Shitty Committee 24/7.

LISTEN TO YOUR CHEERLEADER

Now it's time to hand the mic over to your inner Wise Cheerleader and feel what it's like when you have that voice in your head, following you around all day.

I mean, just imagine it. With this voice whispering in your ear the majority of the time, you'd find yourself wanting to fill your days doing the things you enjoy, you'd prioritize your well-being and happiness, you'd be drawn to the people, the work, the activities and the places that make you come alive. You'd surround yourself with people that make you feel loved and respected and move away from the people that don't. You'd have the courage to speak your truth and make a stand for what you believe in. You'd listen to your dreams and turn them into projects to bring them to life. You'd be coming from a place of love and welcome it into your life.

And, when the pressure is on because work has intensified, you're on a tight deadline or you're suddenly having to spin a million and one plates, your inner Wise Cheerleader would have you pull out all the self-care tools that you have to help you stay calm and focused. You'd ask for help, get plenty of rest and keep yourself hydrated and moving. You'd look after yourself *really well*.

Rather than slipping into overdrive and into your burn-out archetype, your inner Wise Cheerleader will have you remain in power, playing to your strengths. You will feel able to meet the challenges of the day with confidence and you will thrive.

MAKE IT HAPPEN

Wouldn't it be great to have *that* voice accompanying you throughout your day and throughout your life?

Well you *can* have that.

Because you *do* have that wise supportive voice inside of you. Just think of how you speak to your friends and the people you love.

The problem is, while we all happily speak to our friends with love, kindness and compassion, for most people, the idea of speaking to themselves in this way sounds totally alien. Cringey even... until they try it.

Learning to speak to yourself with love and respect is a radical act. Because of the huge impact it has on your life when you do.

If you focused *only* on cultivating that friendly, supportive inner voice for the next year, so that it became the dominating voice in your life, that alone would have the power to transform your life, *in every* area.

Write a letter to yourself from your wise 80-year-old self

To cultivate your own inner Wise Cheerleader you have to practise speaking to yourself with love, kindness and support. One of the most powerful ways to do that is to write letters or messages of love and support to you from you, because no one knows better than you what words you need to hear. And, when you relax, set your mind free and allow the words to just come out on the page, you'll often find you give yourself some pretty wise advice.

I've been doing this for years and I LOVE it – it is so surprisingly powerful.

Imagine that you are receiving a letter from your wise older self (you can also imagine you're receiving the letter from someone you admire, an ancestor, a higher power, whatever works for you). This deeply loving and supportive version of you is reaching back to the person you are today, looking upon you with so much love and with so much wisdom to offer. Let that wise version of you write a letter of love and support to you.

Don't over think it, just give it a go.

If a whole letter feels too big a leap right now, then write yourself a couple of lines of love and motivation on a post-it. Writing 'you've got this' on a post-it always gives me a boost of confidence. And I know that might sound crazy when that vote of support is coming from you and not someone else. But I promise you, *it works*.

Knowing how to turn down the volume on your Shitty Committee and how to turn up the volume on your inner Wise Cheerleader are two of the most essential tools that you'll need to help you start thriving in life.

You'll find these tools coming up a lot as we go through the rest of the book. So keep them by your side as we dive into the rest of the tool kit that will help you go from exhausted and burnt out to feeling like you have more energy than you ever thought possible.

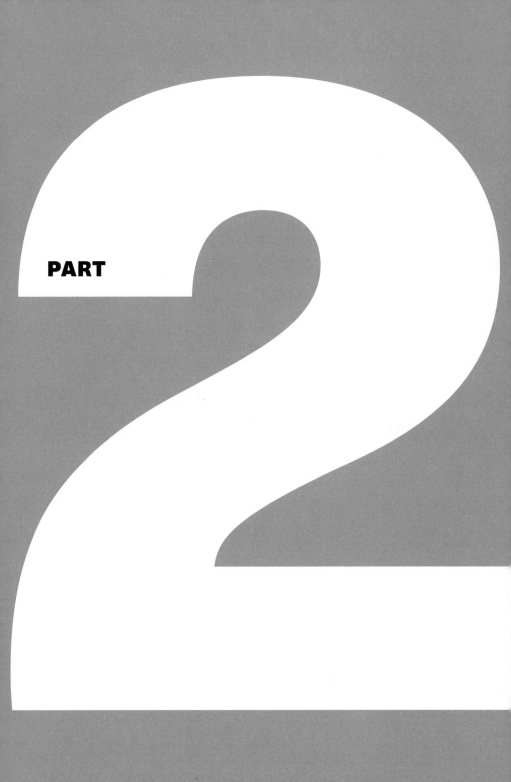

PART

2

RECLAIM YOUR ENERGY

Burnout is, in a nutshell, one big human energy crisis. Being tired, worn out and exhausted seems to be the new modern day normal. Even when we're not burning out, many of us experience a relentless lack of energy, and not just on the physical level. We are overdrawn and bankrupt on every energy level: physical, emotional, mental and spiritual.

We all know that you can't spend your life running on empty, but we seem unable to do it any other way. Our natural energy and vitality has gone. And we need to get it back. If we're going to thrive in this fast-paced digital world, we need to become masters at managing our own energy – Olympic-athlete style.

Discovering how to manage my energy totally changed my life. After years of constant fatigue and mini burnouts, today I have more energy and vitality than I ever thought was possible. And it feels amazing. Don't get me wrong, I have my off days, my tired days and my meltdowns, but generally, I'm full of energy, which means that I get to be the kind of partner, mother, friend, coach, daughter and sister I want to be. I feel able to go after my dreams without being afraid that I'll burn out again. I wake up in the morning feeling refreshed and energized and manage to feel that way for most of the day.

When life gets tough or the pressure is on, I know I have the energy, the resilience and the tools to cope with it and on a day-to-day basis I get to feel alive and well in my body. And there really is no better feeling than that.

Unlocking the secrets to knowing how to manage my energy on every level has transformed my life. Now I want to show you how you can do it, too.

Physical energy

Physical energy is the primary source of fuel in your life. Without physical energy flowing abundantly, nothing else is going to flow well either – it's like trying to run a car without fuel.

When you're running low on physical energy, life is far more likely to feel like a struggle. Not only does your body feel tired, but you are more likely to feel negative, emotional, foggy, slow, irritable and lacking in confidence and motivation.

When your body is fully alive with physical energy and vitality, you feel alive. You feel strong, motivated and ready to take on the challenges of the day. Nothing beats that feeling.

Whether you are recovering from burnout, tired of being tired all the time or simply wanting to learn how to thrive and be happy in life, learning how to manage your physical energy is always the best place to start.

Let's get physical!

For years I used to dream of having energy and vitality, and I had honestly given up hope of ever having any. I was resigned to the fact that, as a working mother, living among the frenetic pace of London and running my own business, it was inevitable that I was going to feel tired a lot of the time – and probably for most of my life.

Because, you see, I thought human energy worked in the same way that a smartphone works when you go out for the day without your charger; you start the day with a full battery, and over the course of the day you use up your energy, until you arrive home exhausted with just a sliver of battery life remaining.

I thought that the energy you had at the start of the day was all the energy you were going to get. And that the only way you could gain any extra battery was by boosting yourself with coffee or sugar, or both. And so often, I used both.

So, when people told me I should exercise, I told them through gritted teeth that I didn't have the time or energy to exercise. I was using up my energy on other more urgent things, thank you very much, like earning a living and caring for a child.

I thought they didn't get it. But it turns out that I didn't get it. The truth was I had no idea how my body worked. I had no idea how to manage my energy. I had no idea that I *could* manage my energy.

When I finally discovered that I could charge myself up with energy whenever I needed it – that I could start the day full of energy and end the day still full of energy – it changed my life.

Finally, after years of feeling tired from the moment I woke up to being exhausted by the time I hit my bed, I become one of those mythical people that was full of energy and vitality.

I felt like I'd won the lottery. Learning how to fill myself up with physical energy and keep it topped up throughout the day has honestly been life changing, and I am SO excited to now be finally sharing it with you.

If you dream of not feeling tired for the rest of your life, if you want to feel full of energy and vitality every day, then read on – that possibility is entirely within your reach.

If *I* can go from tired *all* of the time *for years*, to feeling energized most of the time, then so can you.

So, let's do it!

FUEL YOURSELF

We all know that what we eat and drink affects our energy levels. That we need to drink plenty of water to stay hydrated (dehydration is a huge energy drain) and eat nourishing food to keep ourselves energized and fuelled throughout the day. But do you actually do that? Particularly on the days when the pressure is on and you have a hundred and one other things to do.

There's a reason that a lot of us fail to fuel ourselves properly on busy, full-on days.

Because when you're in fight-or-flight mode, you are less connected to your body and what it needs.

It's a deliberate tactic by your body so that you can be fully focused on surviving the threat to your life (even if that threat is actually just a tight deadline).

Then when stress hormones have been running through your body for some time, you'll find yourself craving sugar and foods high in fat, which can work in the short term to reduce stress and give you an energy boost but, after the initial spike in energy, you're likely to come crashing down, which throws your body back into fight or flight.

On top of that, when you're feeling as if you're competing against the clock, you can often feel that you simply don't have the time to stop and eat a proper meal. You end up barely making time for a bathroom break.

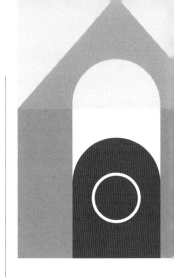

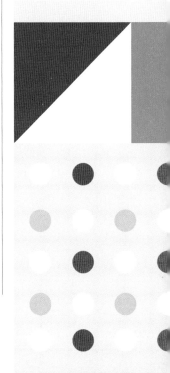

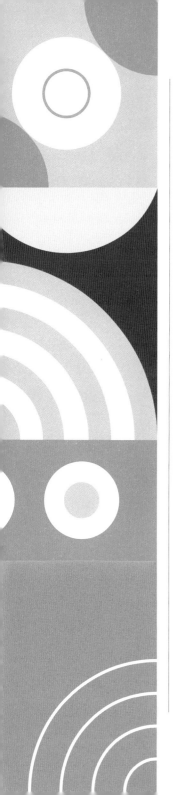

So it's all too easy to find yourself reaching for fast-food, sugar and caffeine to get you through the day. And this is not the way to fuel your body.

The key is to first learn what food and drink really helps fuel your body during the day, then make it as easy and effortless as possible for you to eat those foods, particularly on the full-on days.

Now, I'm not going to tell you what you should or shouldn't eat. What you eat is up to you.

I'm a big fan of intuitive eating – eating what feels right to you and your body and not restricting yourself. So, if you don't know yet what food and drinks really energize you, experiment. Some experts recommend six small meals a day to keep your energy levels topped up, while other experts suggest that our energy reserves should be deeper and that snacks shouldn't be necessary. You might find that including complex carbohydrates for breakfast, such as oats, is just what you need to feel focused all morning or you might run better on protein such as eggs or yoghurt.

Eat right

One of the biggest problems with our eating habits is the ease of junk food and processed foods. So, the key is to make the good stuff easy and to hand.

Ways you can do this:

- Eat the same nourishing breakfast every day so you don't even have to think about it.
- Always have a bowl of fruit or nuts (or whatever is a nourishing snack for you) to hand and keep it topped up so that you can reach for it when you need a snack.
- Take a homemade lunch into work or identify the cafes and shops near where you work that offer you nourishing lunch options that you enjoy.
- Keep a water bottle on hand and topped up for staying hydrated throughout the day. It's the absolute best pick-me-up for a tired or frazzled mind.
- Pick out 5–10 meals that you know you love to eat and make sure you always have the ingredients for at least three of them in your kitchen so that it is easy for you to create. Don't know what your top 5–10 meals are? Do some exploring and experimenting. Read some of the billions of recipe books out there that show you how to make the food you love and find your favourites.
- Batch cook food on the weekend so you have food to eat during the week that you don't need to prep. Just warm it up and eat.

And finally, if you are really into coffee, which I am, what I've found helps to stop it from becoming an unhealthy habit is to be mindful of how I'm using it. If I'm reaching for a coffee from a place of pleasure, then I'm good to go, but if I'm reaching for it out of a need for energy that I'm lacking, then I just ask myself, what else I can do to give myself that energy boost? and I make sure I give myself that – it could be a 20-minute break, food, fresh air or a yogic coffee (see page 75). And, sometimes, I still have the coffee (with a glass of water on the side). The key is, make sure you don't use coffee, sugar or any other stimulants, as an artificial energy booster, because you can slip pretty quickly into your overdrive mode.

MOVE YOUR BODY

Possibly one of the most annoying things you could have once said to me when I was tired was, 'You should go and do some exercise.'

How, if I already felt physically exhausted, was exercise going to help? Surely it would take away even *more* energy from me. Energy that I didn't have. Not to mention it would also use up time that I didn't have.

And so, it is with a deep sigh that I am now having to sit here and tell you the following:

If you seem to be spending your life feeling tired and lacking in energy, then there is one big thing that is going to make an enormous difference. (I can't tell you how sorry I am to break this to you.)

It's exercise.

Far from depleting your energy, doing exercise GIVES you energy. It charges you up. One of the reasons so many of us are suffering fatigue is that we aren't using our bodies *enough*. We need to get our bodies moving, our hearts pumping and our muscles strengthening and stretching.

If you come home at the end of the day feeling exhausted, with barely any energy to make your own dinner, then do half an hour of exercise and you'll miraculously get your energy back.

Learning this has changed my life.

If you don't currently exercise at all, this is what is going to change your life.

Exercise seems to be hands-down the number one ingredient that has got most people back on their feet after burning out.

Because exercise doesn't just give you more physical energy, it can help boost your emotional and mental energy, too.

It is the key to feeling happier, stronger, more capable, more resilient and better able to cope when things get tough. It helps you to think more positively and increases your confidence while also boosting your self-esteem.

And before you start thinking that doing exercise means having to go to the gym every day, I promise you it doesn't. As long as what you're doing gets your heart pumping, your body moving and your muscles working then it's exercise.

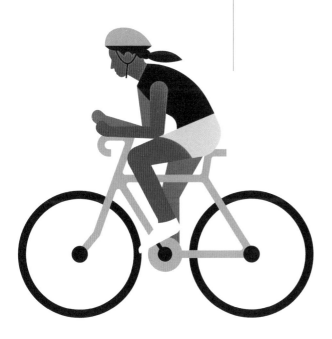

How often should you exercise?

Well, the experts all seem to say pretty much the same thing:

30 minutes of aerobic exercise (getting your heart pumping) three times a week.

As long as you're doing something that gets your heart pumping and your body moving for half an hour then you can do what you want. You could have mini dance raves in your kitchen, do a HIIT workout in your living room, have some energetic sex, go for a run in the park, lift weights, climb trees, go to a yoga class, hit the gym, mop the kitchen floor. It's up to you.

30 minutes of strength training (strengthening and stretching your muscles) twice a week.

The same applies – all sorts of activities can help you to strengthen your muscles, from lifting weights to yoga, digging in the garden, HIIT workouts, doing squats in your living room. What's important is that you're working the muscles in all the main muscle groups and you need to tire the muscles out.

But, when you're getting started, remember that any amount of regular activity is better than nothing at all. It is not all or nothing. So, if you can only manage 10 minutes twice a week, start there.

If you don't already have forms of exercise that you do regularly that give you an aerobic workout or strengthen and stretch your muscles, then get exploring. Find what works for you, what you enjoy and what is easy to weave into your day and start doing it.

Stretch

As well as exercising, stretching is also an amazing way to get the energy flowing through your body. A great form of stretching is yoga and pilates, but even just a few stretches while sitting at your desk can give you an immediate energy boost, particularly if you sit at a desk all day.

Find ways to weave regular stretching into your day. For example, any time you get up to go to the bathroom, make a cup of tea or get something from the photocopier, use it as an opportunity to stretch.

When you're reading something on your computer, rather than sitting with your hands frozen at the keyboard, use it as a chance to get in a few stretches. It will also naturally have you taking a few deep breaths at the same time.

Just give it a try and you'll soon discover the power stretching has to give you more energy throughout the day.

Check your posture

Your posture affects everything from your energy levels to your ability to focus and concentrate, to your breathing, your organ function and even your mood and mental health.

Sitting slouched at a desk with your shoulders tense and rigid and your head looking down at your computer could be draining your energy more than you realize. So, as well as regular movement and stretching, you need to make sure that your body is comfortable and supported. Poor posture, uncomfortable seating and lack of support can cause pain in your body and make your muscles work harder, which often leads to feelings of tiredness and low energy.

Consider if you need a better chair, a stand for your laptop or even try a standing-up desk.

BREATHE

Breathing is one of the greatest energizers there is – when you do it properly.

The fact is, a lot of us don't breathe well. Which seems bizarre. You'd think that having done it every second from the moment that we were born, we'd be experts at it. But no. And, if you spend a lot of your day sitting down working, the chances are you're pretty bad at it. In fact, sometimes, without realizing it, when you're checking your emails, you might not be breathing at all!

Shallow breathing, which is what a lot of us do, increases our feelings of anxiety and robs us of our energy. What you want to be doing instead is taking slow, deep breaths as much as possible.

Take a moment right now and take a slow, deep breath through your nose counting to four and then exhale through your mouth, slowly counting to six. Do it twice more. Feels good, doesn't it?

The extra oxygen instantly energizes you (which is why we yawn when we're tired), it helps to calm your nervous system when you're stressed, helps you think more clearly and helps you sleep better.

Deep breathing in your day

1. Take three slow, deep breaths regularly throughout the day (try putting a reminder alarm on your phone every hour – it does make a difference).

2. Find ways to get more deep breathing back into your day. Whenever you stand up from your desk or are standing in a queue, use it as a trigger to remind you to roll your shoulders back, stretch out your arms and take in a few slow, deep breaths. It is amazing what a difference it can make to your overall energy levels. You can also find free breathing exercises on YouTube, or look for a 'breath work' class in your local area.

Yogic coffee

There are so many great breathing exercises you can do, but one of my favourites is 'yogic coffee' (also known as *Bhastrika* or 'Bellows Breath'). It's a really easy 30-second breathing exercise that gives you an immediate energy boost – better than an actual coffee.

How to do it: Pump your arms up and down fast while you breathe air in and out of your nose as hard as you can. As you breathe in, stretch your arms up fast. As you breathe out, bring your arms down fast, bending at the elbows so you help squeeze the air out of your body as you gently push your arms into your sides. Now repeat that as fast as you can for 30 seconds. (Search for 'yogic coffee' online for a video demonstration.)

AND... RELAX

I want you to imagine for a moment that you are on holiday, lying in a hammock or floating on the water, listening to the soothing sound of birdsong, wind in the trees, lapping water. Just imagine how relaxed your body would be...

Now that is how relaxed you need your body to feel *every day*, including on a cold, wet, grey winter's day. In fact, *particularly* on those days. Because as much as we need to move our bodies to feel energized, we also need to *relax* our bodies.

Daily physical relaxation helps you to release stress, calm your nervous system, ground yourself, quiet your mind, flood your body with feel-good hormones and get back into your body and the present moment.

It is something a lot of us only let ourselves do when we're on holiday.

That needs to change.

You need to find ways to let your body fully and deeply relax every day. And don't assume you do that in your sleep. Many of us clench our jaws and grind our teeth while we sleep – hardly the sign of a relaxed body.

Activities to help relax your body and mind

- A hot relaxing bath (a hot bath or shower releases oxytocin into the body – the same hormone that is released when you're having an orgasm)
- Massage or a back rub
- Lying in a hammock
- An orgasm
- Breathing exercises
- Yin yoga
- A relaxing guided meditation or visualization
- Yoga nidra
- Tai chi
- Qi gong

Find what works for you and make it a priority in your life.

Allowing yourself to fully and deeply relax can't just be a nice-to-have treat when you feel you deserve it or something you do when you have time. It's an essential daily requirement if you want to feel energized and thrive in life.

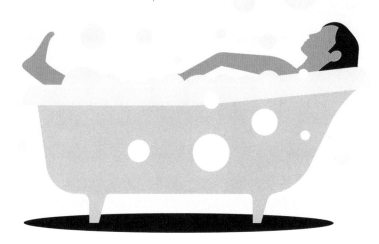

SLEEP

If you're going to get hooked on anything in life, make it sleep.

A good night's sleep is transformative. It is the ultimate rejuvenator and energizer.

When we sleep, our body rests, restores and renews its energy, repairing muscle, organs and other cells, while our brain processes what went on during the day. You can't cheat it. Sleep studies have found that not getting enough sleep impacts negatively on your ability to concentrate, your memory, your IQ and your immune system.

I used to rarely go to bed before midnight, but now I'm in bed every night by 10pm and ideally asleep before 11pm, because when I don't get at least eight hours of sleep a night life just feels harder. I struggle to fully engage in my work, I don't have the energy to run around and play with my son and I don't enjoy my day, I just survive through it.

Sleep has been my saviour since becoming a mother.

Any time I feel like I'm starting to get run down or if I feel as if I've got a cold coming on, early to bed and a good nine to ten hours' sleep nearly always sorts me out.

Sleep is a healer.

But, when you're burnt out or heading into burnout, while you might feel exhausted during the day, it can often be difficult to sleep at night, particularly if you're an over-thinker who struggles to switch off at the best of times. You can find yourself feeling so wired that you struggle to get to sleep and so anxious that you struggle to stay asleep. Insomnia is a very common burn-out symptom.

If sleep is something you struggle with, then here are a few things that can help:

- Go to bed at the same time every night
- Switch your phone and screens off at least half an hour before bedtime
- Have a hot bath to deeply relax your body
- Use essential oils to help you feel relaxed and sleepy
- Drink a herbal tea that will help you fall asleep
- Write a gratitude list (studies have shown that it improves sleep)
- Write out any thoughts that are going round your head that might keep you awake
- Read before you go to bed
- Meditate or listen to yoga nidra before you go to bed
- Listen to stories or a sleep meditation to help you fall asleep
- Breathe in slowly for a count of four and out for six to help you get to sleep
- Bring the temperature of your room down to 18°C (64°F) – the ideal sleeping temperature, apparently
- Give alcohol a break – this can be a big one – I've seen a lot of people transform their sleep (and energy levels) quite literally overnight by cutting out alcohol

To really get you in the mood for sleep, you could also try the activities on how to relax your body (see page 77) or the Stress SOS steps to help to calm your nervous system (see pages 96–7). If you have trouble switching your mind off from work, see the tips on page 193.

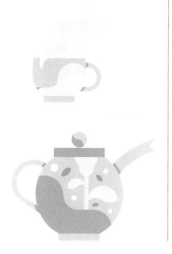

If you are often woken up by an anxious mind that seems to think that 1am, 3am and 5am are ideal times to try and solve all your life and work problems, try the following:

- Something that normally helps you to get to sleep – a breathing exercise, meditation, yoga nidra or a sleep-time story
- If you've got ideas racing around in your mind, try writing them all down to get them out of your head
- If, after 15–20 minutes, you still can't get to sleep, get up and out of bed. It's important that you don't start thinking of your bed as a place where you struggle to get to sleep as that will only make it worse. So instead get up and do something calming and relaxing until you feel sleepy again and can fall back into bed and back to sleep

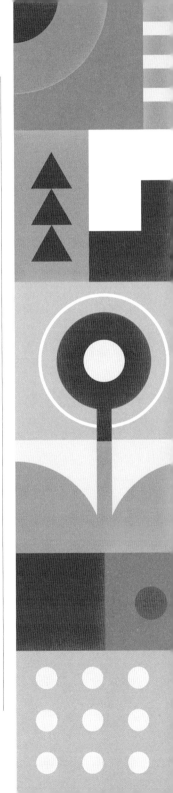

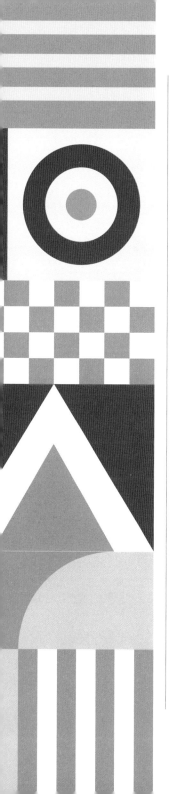

RECOVER

No matter how good you are at looking after yourself, sometimes you are going to use up all your energy and wear yourself out. Whether that's from pulling a couple of long days and late nights to meet a deadline (writing this book certainly involved a few towards the end!), having a wild weekend with a lot of partying or travelling regularly for work.

When you do feel worn out, make sure you book in recovery time afterwards so that you can rest, relax and fully recharge your batteries. Really dedicate time to it and take your recovery seriously.

Have fun, nap, relax, have hot baths. Do things that help release any built-up stress (see page 194) and that 'fill up your cup' (see page 133). Why not treat yourself to a digital detox to give yourself some time unplugged from the rest of the world (see page 120)?

FIND YOUR RHYTHM

As human beings, we are naturally rhythmic creatures.

From our 24-hour circadian inner clock, to our rhythmic sleep pattern and the menstrual cycle (for those of us that have one), we are dictated by the natural cycles and rhythms within us, while being equally affected by the cycles and rhythms around us, from the seasons to the position of the moon to the rising and setting of the sun.

Under the influence of these cycles and rhythms in and around us, our energy ebbs and flows throughout the day, the month and the year as naturally as the tide goes in and out, pulled by the moon.

As Tony Schwartz and Jim Loehr, authors of *The Power of Full Engagement* and my absolute Obi Wans when it comes to energy management, say, 'We are oscillatory beings in an oscillatory universe. Rhythmicity is our inheritance.'

Once upon a time, we used to live in sync with the pulse and natural rhythms of life within us and around us. Living in this rhythmic way is what kept us energized. We used our energy and we renewed it as naturally as the sun rises and sets. But, we don't live like that anymore. Instead, we treat ourselves as if we are a machine – pushing on through, keeping ourselves going 24/7, ignoring our body's natural call to rest and recharge our batteries on a regular basis.

So, in order for each of us to reclaim our energy, we need to get back into a rhythmic way of living. Because when we do, we'll get our energy back and our lives back.

Get back in sync with the natural rhythms

The circadian rhythm is your 24-hour inner biological clock that matches the earth's 24-hour cycle. Things that throw your circadian rhythm out of whack are night shifts, jet lag and going to bed and getting up at different times each day. For optimal energy, you need to get in sync with your circadian rhythm.

Here is how you can do it:

- Stick to a regular sleep schedule: go to bed and get up at the same time every day (give or take 30 minutes)
- Avoid looking at screens before bed
- Get outside every morning
- Sleep in a cool, dark room (invest in an eye mask, or thick curtains or blinds for the summer months)
- Be prepared for the mid-afternoon drop in energy. Your circadian rhythm is the cause of those mid-afternoon slumps in energy – a natural energy dip around 1–4pm. To combat it, have a nap, go for a walk or dance around to help renew your energy

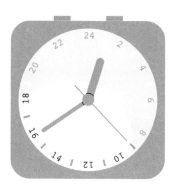

Night owls and morning larks

Some of us are natural larks and like to get up early and leap into the day, and others are natural night owls and find that we enjoy working later into the night. This is a result of your own personal circadian rhythm, known as your chronotype. Larks naturally wake up early and go to bed early, and their energy levels are at their optimum in the morning. Night owls naturally wake up later and go to bed later, and their energy levels are usually at an optimum in the evening.

The problem is when you try to fit into a schedule that doesn't suit your natural circadian rhythm.

A 9–5pm working schedule can be a struggle for night owls, who hit their energy peak after 5pm, as well as for larks who naturally hit their peak before 9am.

If you enjoy a flexible work schedule, then ditch the traditional 9–5pm approach and set a work schedule that works for you. If you can't do that, leave the work that requires your greatest focus and brain power for the times in the day when you are closest to your energy peak.

If you're a lark, get into the heavy-duty work first thing in the morning and leave the light tasks for the afternoon and night owls should do the light tasks in the morning when you're still waking up and leave the deep-focused work for later in the afternoon or evening.

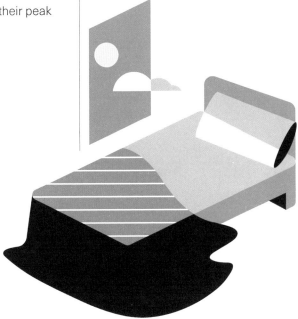

The monthly cycle

If you have a menstrual cycle, your energy levels and mood will vary throughout your cycle. When you're ovulating, you will find you have a lot more energy and desire to be out and about in the world. This is called the summer of your cycle.

When menstruating, you'll be feeling at your lowest ebb when it comes to energy (and sometimes mood), but at your most intuitive. This is called the winter of your cycle and it's a time for rest, reflection and hibernation. When you start to understand how your menstrual cycle affects you, you can start to plan what activities to focus on, depending on what 'season' you are in, so that you can optimize your natural energy levels.

I have seen women's lives transform when they start to work in harmony with their menstrual cycle. *In the FLO* and *WomanCode* by Alisa Vitti are great books to consult for more information.

Seasonal changes

Many of us find that our energy levels are also strongly affected by the seasons. The lack of daylight during the winter months naturally leaves us with less energy and many of us feel the desire to hibernate and go to bed earlier. Meanwhile, in the spring and summer months many of us will find we have a lot more energy, want to be outside more and go to bed later. Again, allow yourself to sync with this natural rhythm. In the winter, spend more time snuggling, resting, reflecting and enjoying hygge activities – making things, cooking, having deep talks with a warm drink in your hands. In the summer, get outdoors, go on adventures, meet new people and make things happen.

If in the winter months, you struggle from SAD (Seasonal Affective Disorder), getting as much natural daylight as you can, regular exercise and a SAD lamp to brighten your day can help to raise your energy levels and your mood.

LISTEN TO YOUR BODY

If you really want to thrive in life, then you need to start listening to your body.

Really listening. Your body knows what you need to feel energized. It is wise and it is smart. Too many of us live from the neck up, ignoring our bodies and what they are communicating to us.

When you stop overriding your body, start listening to it and do as it says, you will naturally return to balance and vitality. But reconnecting to your body and learning how to listen to it takes time. Start by checking in with your body throughout the day. Tune in to find out if it is thirsty or hungry. When your body says it needs a rest, have a rest. When you start to feel run down and exhausted, get an early night or spend the following weekend really resting, relaxing and recharging your batteries.

Breaking out of the burn-out cycle is largely about returning to your body and remembering what it is to thrive. Your body already knows, it's for you to learn to listen.

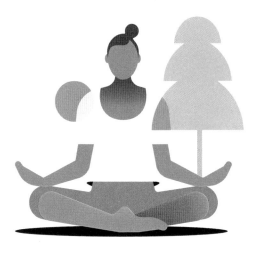

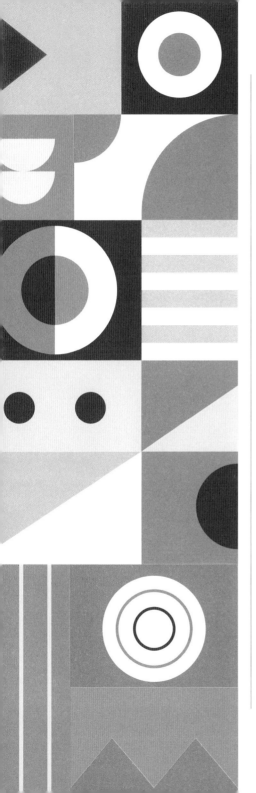

What do you need to do right now?

- Which of the key steps to keeping your body energized (see pages 66–86) do you feel most in need of right now or which one is calling to you the most?
- What do you need to do to make that happen?
- What is the next step you will take to do that?

_____
_____
_____
_____
_____
_____
_____
_____
_____
_____
_____
_____
_____
_____
_____
_____

Mental
energy

One of the biggest causes of burnout is *mental* burnout. You know when it hits – it feels like a fuse has gone in your brain, suddenly even the simplest of decisions can seem overwhelming.

You feel frazzled, too exhausted to think, but too wired to be able to fall asleep. You want to switch off but you're not sure you know how. You can feel anxious and worn out or overwhelmed and depressed. You struggle to focus, your brain feels slow and sluggish. It's as if your brain has gone on strike. And maybe it has. Maybe it *should*.

The fact is, our brains were not designed for the modern world. From the speed at which we are having to process new information, to the constant demands of our smart phones, to a working day that runs for eight hours+ with, at best, a one-hour break in the middle – we are asking way too much of our poor brains.

This is not how to make the most of our powerful, and frankly, magical, minds.

Our overworked minds

At best, we treat our minds like machines, at worst, like slaves. We have them managing our to-do lists, processing a never-ending stream of information, constantly asking them to make decisions and reassess plans and schedules.

We have them forever jumping from one task to the next, often asking them to attempt multiple tasks at the same time while simultaneously keeping an eye on the time, our email inbox and any notifications of new messages that might have popped up.

We are so conditioned by the post-industrial work culture that treats people like machines, that we do the same to our own minds, never considering that they need a rest, thinking that we can keep them switched on 24/7, forcing them to operate from an almost-permanent state of fight or flight and then wondering why we are feeling so stressed out and exhausted all the time.

'I'll rest later', we think. But later never comes. Instead we keep pushing on, keep piling things onto our plates, driving ourselves forward on adrenaline, thinking that *this* is the only way we're going to get through that enormous to-do list and hit those pressing deadlines. Thinking that this is what productivity looks like.

It's not. This is what chronic stress and inefficiency looks like.

Your work suffers, your brain suffers, your relationships suffer and you suffer. And when you're in that state, it feels like there is no way out. But I promise you – there is.

Just like your body, your brain is designed to thrive. It is designed to be calm, alert, engaged, present and focused. But, a fast-moving frenetic, noisy, distracting, always-on digital modern world does not provide your brain with the conditions it needs to be that way. Quite the opposite.

And so in order for you to give your brain what it needs to thrive, you need to learn how to unplug from the high-speed, stressed-out adrenalized pace of the modern working world, declutter your life of all the unnecessary daily stressors that throw your brain into a state of panic and distress, and learn how to set your mind free and give it the conditions it needs to get it back in flow and to its full power.

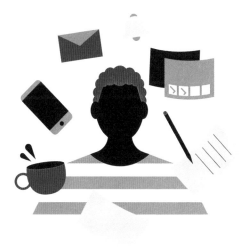

Let's talk about stress

It's time to finally mention the elephant in the room. The reason why we're all here and why so many of us are burning out: stress.

Stress has become a modern-day obsession. We say we don't want to be stressed. We claim we want stress-free lives, but at the same time we *expect* our lives to be stressful. We're told that this is just how modern life is. That life in this day and age is more stressful than it has ever been. And so, just like with our incessant busyness, we wear our stress like a badge of honour. We seek it out because we think it's a sign that we are hardworking, successful and at our most productive. And it's expected of us.

Most managers and CEOs, whether they admit it or not, like to see their teams speeding around the place, jacked up on adrenaline, busying away non-stop because they, too, believe that this is how you get the most done in the fastest time. If those CEOs and managers were to suddenly see their teams looking calm, relaxed and taking regular breaks at work, I bet they would start to worry that their teams weren't dedicated enough, working hard enough or being productive enough.

But, living in such high levels of stress is making us ill, making us miserable and making us burnout. The problem is, in our messed-up, modern work culture this kind of frantic, panicked, urgent stress has been confused for being a sign of dedication, caring about your work and having important things to do. We've been programmed to think that we have to be that stressed to get through the day and generate the energy to get all the things done, but actually when you're in that stressed-out state, you are at your least productive, least effective and least efficient.

What happens when you're stressed out:

- Your IQ drops
- You are unable to think clearly, rationally, intuitively or creatively
- You are prone to making mistakes
- You are irritable
- You are much slower at your work
- You get tunnel vision and can no longer see the big picture or get any perspective on things
- You naturally start to think and feel more negative than usual
- Your motivation drops
- You start to doubt your abilities
- The volume goes up on your Shitty Committee

STRESS – THE GOOD KIND

Contrary to popular belief, stress isn't all bad. In fact, the idea that we should be aiming for a stress-free life is totally wrong. A stress-free life would be a stagnant and disengaged life. Basically, a bit meh – no enthusiasm, no excitement, no fire in your belly. You'd be buffeted along by life, never fully engaging, never going after your dreams, never realizing your potential and never growing.

Here is the thing about stress: we do actually need stress in our lives, not just to survive, but to thrive. But what we need is the right kind of stress. The good stress, otherwise known as eustress.

The stress that most of us are running on is *distress*.

Yes, there are two different kinds of stresses, each with equally important roles in our lives.

DISTRESS: The panicky 'a tiger is chasing me!!!' kind of stress where you either play dead or run as fast as you can.

EUSTRESS: The exhilarating 'yikes this is a challenge, but I can do it' kind of stress where you rise to the challenge and feel in flow.

Distress is essential when a hungry tiger is heading towards you, when your house is burning down or when your child is about to run into oncoming traffic.

You could not ask for a better companion in that moment. This powerful fight-or-flight response is quite literally a lifesaver. However, that kind of stress is the 'break in case of emergency' kind of stress. It should only be used in a very real life-threatening emergency, but, in the modern work environment, we're in this state a *lot* of the time.

In our fast-paced, pressurized, highly visible, socially complex modern world, everything feels urgent or feels like a threat, such as:

- Looming deadlines
- Getting to a meeting on time
- Making a good impression
- Not messing up
- Not looking like an idiot
- Being liked
- Not being rejected
- Getting praised and validated
- Not failing

… the list of potential threats to our survival is endless. Our Shitty Committee is run off its feet, and the over-giver, over-doer, over-thinker and over-achiever are all out in full force.

In this high-stress environment, cortisol can be pumping through your body almost continuously, suppressing your immune system, pushing you into burnout and, in the long term, increasing your risk of cancer and auto-immune diseases. We simply weren't designed to be in this distressed state so much of the time. And it's making us ill.

Eustress, on the other hand, is actually *good* for you.

Eustress energizes and motivates you; it feels exciting, it increases your focus and performance, engages your full attention and helps you to rise to the challenge. In its best form, eustress can induce a state of flow – that state of mind where you feel totally and utterly absorbed in the moment.

Think about a time when you have felt really fired up about a project, whether it was at work or not. As you worked on it, you felt excited, you enjoyed the momentum and pace of it and you were fully absorbed, engaged and calm. It felt challenging in a fun and exhilarating kind of way. That is eustress. And *that* is the kind of stress you want when the pressure is on at work. For this to happen you need to learn how to shift the gears out of *di*stress and into *eu*stress. Which means shifting out of an urgent, panicked, stressed-out state that is fuelled by fear, and into an alert, fully engaged, fired-up state fuelled by a 'can-do' attitude.

And to do that, you need to know how to calm your nervous system and turn down the volume on your Shitty Committee.

Stress SOS

Here is a six-step process to help you calm your nervous system the next time you feel yourself starting to slip into a state of (di)stress.

Step 1: Breathe

Take three slow deep breaths, counting in for four and counting out for six. If you can, stretch your arms out wide and high into the sky to really help deepen your breathing and release the stress in your body. This will help to calm your nervous system and cool you down.

If you're really stressed out, you might need a bit more to help calm down. Movement is key when it comes to releasing stress: go for a walk, dance around, shake your body, do some exercise. You'll find a list of different things that can help you to release the day's stresses over on page 194.

Step 2: Express it

Write the stress out on a page, talk the stress out into a voice note or ask a willing friend or colleague to just listen to you as you freak out and get it off your chest.

- I'm panicking that...
- I'm afraid that...
- I'm worried that...

And keep taking those slow deep breaths as you do that.

Talking or writing something down and just acknowledging your fears and how you're feeling can help you get perspective and calm you down further.

Step 3: Challenge your Shitty Committee

Once you're feeling calmer, get curious and ask yourself what your Shitty Committee might be saying that could be throwing you into a panic. What limiting beliefs could it be feeding you right now? Use the exercise on page 46 to challenge those beliefs and turn down the volume on that panicky inner critic.

Step 4: Get practical

Once no longer stuck in a panicked fight-or-flight mode, you'll find you'll be able to think more clearly and practically about what you can actually do.

- Can you let someone know how you feel and how you're being impacted?
- Can you ask for help?
- Can you reassess your goals?
- Can you give yourself some more time?
- Do you need to cancel some plans to give you some space?
- Do you need to take a break?
- Do you need to get some advice?
- Do you need to ask for support?

Step 5: If you need help, get help

If you're struggling to stay calm, to get perspective on things or figure out what to do, then *call a friend*. I can't tell you the number of times I've stressed and stewed and freaked out for hours, days sometimes, until finally I've sent out smoke signals and a friend, partner or colleague has come to my aid and within no time at all has helped calm me down or picked me up off the floor and helped me to get back on track with some loving support and practical advice. So never, ever be afraid to reach out when you're freaking out. It's not always easy to do because you might, like me, want to seem like the person that has it all together but, you know what, your friends are usually delighted to finally be able to help you out.

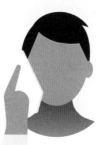

Free yourself from your smart phone

As well as learning how to handle your stress, it's also important to reduce unnecessary stressors in your life. You don't want to spend your whole day doing breathing exercises, shaking and journalling to handle the constant stress triggers coming your way. And modern life is jam-packed with unnecessary stressors. Two of the biggest culprits are smart phones and your to-do list. So, let's start with those.

All over the world, research is being carried out studying the modern person's relationship with their smartphone. From the UK to Brazil and from USA to India, all the research is saying the same thing: we are hooked.

About 80 per cent of us check our phones within 15 minutes of waking up. We then go on to spend about 3 hours on our phones every day, interacting with them, on average, every 12 minutes. We touch our phones (typing, tapping, swiping) on average 2,600 times a day. And then when the day is done, 71 per cent of us go to sleep with our phone next to us (or even in bed with us). And 40 per cent even check our phones in the middle of the night.

Think that's extreme? 24 per cent of people have read or replied to a text message during sex and 12 per cent have *made a phone call* during sex!

Smart-phone addiction has become so normalized that most of us are totally unaware that we even have a problem. But if you are overly attached to your smart phone, it could be having a big impact on your energy and your stress levels. It could even be a big contributor to your burnout.

When I kicked my own smart-phone addiction (and I did *not* think I had a problem) it felt life-changing. Within less than a week, I felt more energized, way less stressed and I got my memory back (which felt miraculous).

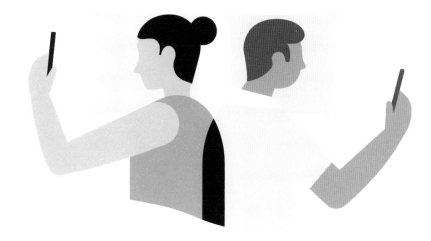

Take this quick test to see if you might be slightly (or very) addicted to your smart phone:

☐ You reach for your phone first thing in the morning.

☐ You spend time on your phone shortly before going to bed most nights.

☐ You immediately pull out your phone when you're feeling bored, have time to kill or are waiting in a queue.

☐ You often fall into a rabbit hole on social media, YouTube or online shopping, mindlessly browsing until you snap back to reality and realize that a good chunk of time has passed by.

☐ You have your phone next to your desk and nearly always check to see what notifications or messages come in as they pop up.

☐ If your phone is in your bag, face down or on silent, you find yourself checking it frequently throughout the day to see if you've got any messages or to check what's happening in the world via the news or social media.

☐ You use your phone when you're working and want a break.

☐ At home you are often found chatting to your family or housemates while also doing stuff on your phone (ask your family and friends to answer that one!).

☐ You feel phantom vibrations – you think your phone has vibrated but when you check, there are no new messages or updates.

☐ You get distressed when you can't find your phone.

☐ When you pop to the shops, even if it's just a 10-minute round trip, you take your phone.

☐ If you were to go out for the day and realized 15 minutes after leaving your house that you'd forgotten your phone, you'd go back to get it, even if it meant being late.

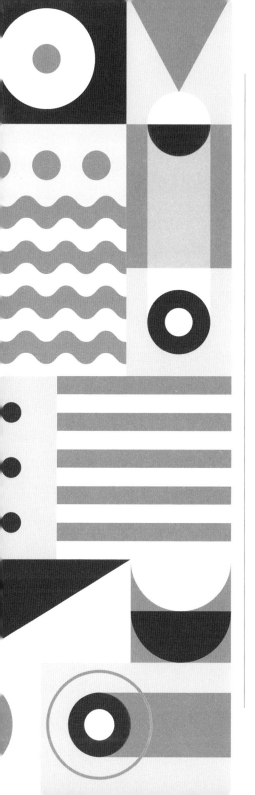

If you ticked two or more, then it's likely you're in a slightly unhealthy relationship with your smart phone.

Not so long ago I would have ticked all the boxes. Which might seem harmless. Scrolling through inspiring content, finding out information or connecting with your friends before bed can't be that bad, right? Making use of those limbo moments with a quick check of your emails – on the train, waiting in the post-office queue, waiting for the kettle to boil – surely that's just being efficient? That might be how it seems, particularly when everyone else is equally attached to their phones, but this is not healthy.

If you have an over-attachment to your smart phone, then it may well be having a much bigger impact on your life than you realize.

Some of the ways that smart-phone addiction affects us

It's trapping us in a 24/7, always available, always-on existence
We are in a new culture of communication where we are expected to be available and open to communication 24/7. Our bosses expect it, as do our clients, our friends, our family. And it's wearing us out.

It's making us stressed...
ALL THE TIME
Every time our phones ping, our bodies get a jolt and release a small level of cortisol, the stress hormone. With messages and alerts popping up on our phones on average every 12 minutes, that cortisol is running through our veins, keeping us in fight-or-flight mode pretty much constantly throughout the day.

It's making us stupid
With all this cortisol running through our bodies, we lose our ability to reflect, think creatively and make decisions. In fact, participants in clinical trials at London's Institute of Psychiatry were found to suffer a 10-point drop in their IQ when they were being distracted by emails and phone calls popping up on their screens.

It's making us WAY less efficient
If you want to get work done fast, the worst thing you can do is have your phone around you. What with the heightened stress levels, the drop in IQ and the constant interruptions, you are undoubtedly less productive and less efficient than you would be if you had your smart phone switched off.

It's playing havoc with our memories
Ever walk into a room and wonder what the hell you went in there to do? It used to happen to me about 20 times a day. A week after I kicked my smart-phone addiction, my memory came back. It was like a flipping miracle.

It's ruining our relationships (and making our kids feel that they're unimportant to us)

It has become socially acceptable to be talking to our friends, colleagues and children while distracted on our phones, which is slowly eating away at the quality of our relationships. A study by AVG Technologies revealed that nearly one-third of children feel unimportant when their parents are on their phones.

It's making us permanently distracted

Sitting with your phone constantly by your side is like having someone sitting next to you whispering your name over and over again, dragging you away from whatever you're doing or who you're with. And don't think that putting it on silent will help. According to research, just knowing that your phone is close by holds you in a state of constant partial attention. It is preventing you from being present to yourself, your life and the people you love.

It's making us feel lonely, depressed and anxious

Despite connecting us to the world and everyone in it, research is proving over and over again that smart-phone addiction leads to an increased rate of depression, anxiety and loneliness.

It's (possibly) making us die sooner

You read that right. Research suggests that overuse of our smart phones could end up shortening our lives, too, because of all the heightened stress we experience because of it.

Don't get me wrong. I love my smart phone. It's a brilliant tool, but it can take over your life, if it hasn't already.

When you start to use your smart phone consciously, rather than mindlessly, it WILL feel like you've got your life back in so many ways. It took me one week to get a handle on my addiction and I couldn't believe the difference it made.

Kicking your smart-phone addiction is like getting a brain upgrade. You'll feel calmer, more focused, more present, happier, less stressed out and, perhaps most magical of all – you'll suddenly get all this extra time. Time you have been craving. Time you have been telling yourself you don't have enough of. It turns out you do – you were just filling it up with your phone.

So, if you're realizing that the way you use your smart phone is an issue, it's time to kick that smart-phone addiction.

Create a new, healthy way of using your smart phone

Turn off all notifications

This is one of the easiest. And while you're at it, turn off all the notifications on your laptop as well. It's bad enough we have our phones pinging incessantly, now we have to have it happening on our laptops too? Stop it. Turn them off.

Take off any social-media apps that are causing anxiety or addictive behaviour

Taking a one-month break from social media that you know you have got addicted to can be a great way to kick the habit. Come back to it more mindfully a month later – when you come back to social media after your break, set yourself clear time boundaries around how often and how long you are going to spend on social media to prevent the addiction from building up again.

Start and end your day phone free

Keep your phone out of your bedroom at night. Get yourself an alarm clock and if you need to charge your phone overnight, place it in another room.

Keep your phone away from your desk when you're working

Having your phone next to you as you work is proven to kill your productivity, your ability to concentrate and your cognitive power. So, turn it off or put it in a drawer. You'll be smarter and more productive as a result.

Stop using your phone when you're bored, need entertaining or are waiting in a queue

It is so important for our minds to be allowed to be idle, to get bored, to ponder, wander and daydream. It is essential for both our creativity and our mental health. But since the arrival of our smart phones, we've stopped allowing our minds this precious time. So, from now on, when you're in one of those natural pauses or rest moments in the day, don't reach for your phone. Instead let your mind wander and go wherever it wants to go. You might be surprised how much you enjoy it.

Be prepared for the withdrawal

The reason we are so obsessed with using our smart phones is because the apps we use on them are designed to get us hooked. So, when you first start reducing the amount of time you use your phone, the chances are you're going to feel it and it isn't going to feel good. My withdrawal was a very real thing. I felt sad and lonely in the first few days. But, I sat it out and, after a few days, the feeling had subsided, and I was free.

Free yourself from your to-do list

Never have our brains been expected to hold the amount of information that they do today.

From the constant flow of news and communications to the ideas, thoughts, decisions that need to be made, the things we are required to remember, plus stuff we're worried about or need to resolve, our minds are in a constant state of high alert just trying to remember everything. And they're not actually very good at it.

As David Allen, author of *Getting Things Done*, says,

'Your brain is designed to come up with ideas, not hold them.'

Your brain can only hold seven (maximum, nine, if you're really good at it) things in your short-term memory at any given time. Seven!

I would happily bet money that you're asking your brain to try to remember a hell of a lot more than seven things at the moment. And if that is the case, that task alone is draining your mental energy and causing you more stress than you might realize.

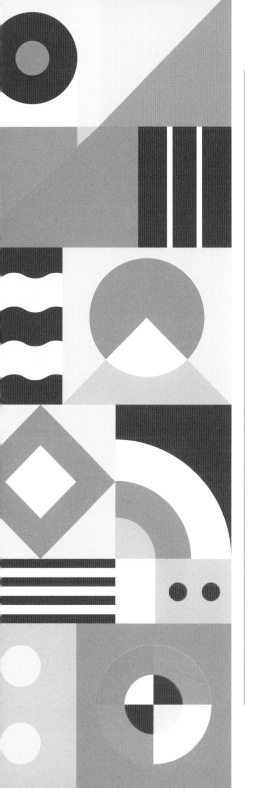

You need to get all of your to-do lists, shopping lists, appointments, meetings and project ideas out of your head (and all the other things you are asking it to remember) on to a page and into a system. A system that you can rely on to tell you what you need to do when you need to do it. Read on to find out how...

Tools to free your mind – and keep it decluttered and organized:

1. A calendar

A calendar that has hourly time slots, where you put in all of your appointments and block out time for different tasks and projects (we'll also be looking at how to use your calendar as your canvas to design your life in Part 3), so that everything you need to do, or projects that you want to spend time on, are given a time and place. No more asking your brain to remember it all.

2. A dedicated place to store your to-do lists

This can be a note app on your phone or on your computer, or an online project management system. Just make sure you know where your lists are so that you can quickly and easily check them and use them to help you keep on top of things. Everything on your to-do list should be in that system and not in your head. Things that have been done need to be ticked off and/or deleted.

3. A dedicated place to keep track of current projects and future project ideas

If you have a lot of different work and home projects that have a lot of moving parts, then you need to have somewhere dedicated to keeping track of them all. Some people love a spreadsheet, some use a project-management system and others like to keep it real with pen and paper. Whatever you use, just make sure you keep them organized and all in one place.

If you get lots of ideas all of the time, keep an ideas bank – a dedicated notebook or document on your phone or laptop where you collect ideas. You don't want to lose those ideas, but you also don't want to use your mental energy by trying to hold on to them.

4. Set a reminder alarm

So that the upcoming appointments and things you have to do today don't keep pulling at your attention, have a reminder alarm that lets you know when it's time to leave for a meeting, make a call or do that task. It can be as simple as an alarm on your phone, a reminder on your laptop or an app on one of your devices. Essentially, it's like having your own personal robot assistant, reminding you of what you need to do so that you don't have to waste time remembering it yourself.

On days when you are feeling overwhelmed and a bit all over the place, check in with yourself and ask, 'What needs to be out of my head, sorted and organized?'

It's much easier to focus and deal with the bigger stuff, when the little stuff is out of your head and dealt with.

You will feel immediately clearer, calmer and back in control. And the same goes for the days or nights when your head is buzzing with anxious thoughts, worries and concerns and preventing you from focusing or falling asleep.

Grab a pen and paper and write down all those thoughts out of your head.

Set that mind of yours free!

Stop multi-tasking (it doesn't work)!

Multi-tasking is a myth.

It drives me nuts that multi-tasking is celebrated as a woman's superpower. It isn't a superpower. You might think you're getting lots of stuff done at the same time, but actually you're just getting lots of things done slowly, and probably badly, because your mind is distracted and jumping around too much. Multi-tasking, by its very nature of making you attempt to handle more than one task at the same time, is a total stressor. On top of that, it has been proven to kill productivity, emotional intelligence, concentration, empathy, self-awareness, attention to detail and lower your IQ. Think of people who check their phones when you're trying to have a conversation with them – they simply aren't in the room. There really is nothing to benefit from multi-tasking.

If you want to reclaim the power of that brain of yours, you need to start doing just *one thing at a time.*

And you might at first need some help in doing that. We have become so used to jumping around rapidly from one task to another (known as task-switching), that many of us have lost our ability to focus and concentrate for any length of time.

The Pomodoro Method

This is a brilliant time-management tool that is designed to help you focus. It is great for those projects that feel overwhelming, for days when you find yourself procrastinating and struggle to focus or when your energy is low. It also has you rhythmically flowing between focused work and rest, so is great for keeping your energy topped up.

The idea is that you decide on what work you're going to focus on and then you set the timer for 25 minutes. When the timer goes off you take a 5-minute break. After the fourth round, you take a longer 15–30-minute break. If you use the Pomodoro method regularly, it helps to train your brain so that over time you should find your focus, attention span and ability to concentrate all improving.

THE THREE-TAB RULE

A tip to stop you from rapid task switching is to try to *only* ever have three tabs open on your desktop at any one time (five, max, if it's absolutely necessary). It helps to keep your mind focused and free from distractions.

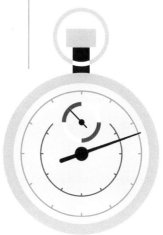

The secret to a happy, calm and powerful mind

Now that we've decluttered your mind and removed many of the unnecessary daily stressors and distractions that have been draining your mental energy and stressing you out, it's time to take a look at what your mind needs in order to truly thrive.

EXERCISE

Again?! Yep. As well as being essential for physical energy, exercise is essential for mental energy and key for mental health. In fact, according to neuroscientist Wendy Suzuki, 'Exercise is the most transformative thing you can do for your brain.'

One workout helps you to renew your mental energy, release stress, clear your mind and boost your confidence and mood. Over time, exercise can help you to build resilience, improve your concentration and has been proven to help protect you from brain deterioration as you grow older. When you're doing a lot of mental labour, one of the best things you can do to help keep your brain from frazzling is exercise. If you're an over-thinker, exercise can be a lifesaver.

When I'm feeling brain frazzled, nothing works better than doing exercise to shake off the stress, get me out of my head and feeling clear-headed and energized again. Try it next time you feel overwhelmed or stressed out. It works like magic!

REST

If there is one thing we need in our society, it's a rest revolution. We are so obsessed with progress, productivity, action and keeping busy that rest is looked upon as, at best, a treat and something you do when you have time and, at worst, an inconvenience – something that if you're strong enough, you can do without. This dismissive way of treating rest is one of the reasons so many of us are suffering from anxiety, overwhelm and burnout.

We have to stop treating rest as 'nice-to-have', and recognize its power as a key, and essential, ingredient to thriving in life.

It's only when you allow your mind to rest that you give it a chance to recharge and renew its energy. And not only that, but when you allow your mind to rest and switch off from using the left side of the brain, where all the day-to-day, rational thinking occurs, you move naturally into the right side of the brain, where all the intuitive thinking, creativity and magic happens.

It's this right side of the brain where all those light bulb moments, sudden insights and intuitive leaps come from. That's why your best ideas usually come to you when you're in the shower, doing exercise, doodling on a notepad, gazing out of the window or washing the dishes. Because you are allowing the left side of your brain to rest and the right side of your brain to do its thing. All the great artists, philosophers, writers, thinkers and scientists know this – they all recognize the power of your unconscious mind.

Einstein once said that, 'The intuitive mind is a sacred gift and the rational mind is a faithful servant. We have created a society that honors the servant and has forgotten the gift.' When you learn to switch off and rest your mind, you get back the gift and power of your intuitive mind. You also get back your energy.

Take a break every 90 minutes

Our bodies are naturally designed to take intermittent rest throughout the day to renew and recharge our batteries.

In fact, we have a brilliant in-built system called our ultradian rhythm, which naturally divides our day into high- and low-frequency brain activity (periods of activity and rest). If we get in sync with it, this ultradian rhythm naturally has us alternating between focused activity and rest.

During the period of high-frequency brain activity you are at your smartest and most alert. This is the perfect time to get focused and dive into your work. After about 90 minutes you'll naturally start to yawn, feel hungry and your brain will feel like it has slowed down. This is a sign that you have moved into a period of lower-frequency brain activity and is a natural signal that it is time to take a break. Your body is literally winding down into rest mode, and it will naturally sit in this state for about 20 minutes.

When this happens, you have a choice:

1. Listen to your body and take a break so that you can renew your energy
2. Over-ride your body's signal that it's time to rest and try to push on through (even though your brain is now no longer firing on all cylinders)

Many of us might be tempted to push on through when we have a lot to do. Pushing on through might feel like the most productive thing to do, but it's not. As countless studies have proven, those of us who don't take breaks are a lot less productive than our colleagues who take a break every 1–2 hours. This is because when you don't stop to renew your energy, you start running on empty, and when that happens your stress levels go up, your IQ drops, you're more prone to making mistakes and you find it harder to focus and think clearly.

So, taking a break from your work every 90 minutes or so, to renew and refresh your energy, isn't just a nice-to-have, it is absolutely essential if you want to do your best work and not wind up stressed out and exhausted at the end of every day.

By plugging into your natural ultradian rhythm and scheduling 20 minute breaks into your working day every 90 minutes or so you will find that you have a lot more energy throughout the day, be able to focus for longer, be more productive, smarter, be able to think more clearly, be a lot less stressed out and happier. It is an instant game changer. Give it a try and just see the difference it makes.

SWITCH OFF FROM WORK

How easy do you find it to switch off from work and let your mind rest?

I mean *really* switch off. Do you find it easy to leave your work behind you at the end of your working day? Do you happily take a break from your work emails and social media when you're on holiday? Do you easily forget about work over the weekend and let yourself get totally absorbed in the present, in activities that bring you pleasure and joy, without finding yourself also quickly checking your emails, catching up on just a few things or simply *thinking* about work? Because I sure as hell do not.

I went for years without ever switching off from work. I would do work on holidays, on the weekend and in bed at night. And even if I wasn't *doing* work, I was *thinking* about it. My big fear was that if I switched off, I might lose my momentum, lose my drive. I was worried that if I slowed down and switched off, I wouldn't be able to gear up again.

Actually, the truth was that I couldn't switch off. I was addicted to my work, addicted to being busy and addicted to the adrenaline that I fuelled myself with to keep myself going during the day so I could work without having to take a break or waste precious time (or at least that is how I saw it). I had been hitting the overdrive button for so long that I couldn't switch myself off any more.

While I'm much better at it now, I *still* find it hard. And I'm not alone. In a world where technology now not only allows us, but encourages us, to be switched on and available all the time, switching off is increasingly hard for people to do. Whether it's switching off from work, social media, from the news or from what our friends are up to.

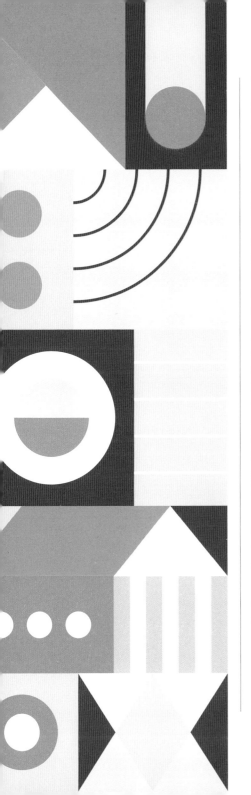

This inability to switch off is making us miserable, wearing us out and, for many of us, it is a big reason for our burnout.

When you are forever switched on, your mind is in a permanent low level state of fight or flight, kept tense and alert by the stress hormones running through your veins, never allowing you to fully relax or let your mind wander and be free, only be distracted, exhausted and disconnected.

A lot of us attempt to use TV, alcohol or drugs to help us switch off. A glass of wine in the evening, Netflix in bed or partying with friends on the weekend. But this isn't real switching off. It's numbing and escapism. It doesn't bring you back to yourself, it doesn't bring you back into the present. And it doesn't allow your body and mind to rest and recharge.

I'm not saying there is anything wrong with having a glass of wine, Netflix in bed or partying on the weekend with friends. I like to do all of those things, but when they become THE way you cope with the stresses of work, then it can become a problem.

Taking your mind off work

The key to switching off is to do things that fully engage your attention and take your mind off work or whatever is occupying your thoughts.

You'll already know some things that work for you, but have some fun exploring and experimenting, discovering what helps you to switch off and get into the right side of your brain:

- Getting out in nature
- Exercise / sport
- Yoga
- Meditation
- Dance
- Martial arts
- Creative activities (such as painting, drawing, pottery, cooking, playing or making music, woodwork, making things, sewing, knitting, crafts, colouring in, making a mandala, doodling)
- Listening to music
- 'Wax-on-wax-off' seemingly mundane activities – anything that has you using your hands or body and engaging in meditative, rhythmic, repetitive motion (such as painting a fence, cleaning the windows, washing up, digging a flower bed)

JUST HIT STOP

It's not always just work that we need to switch off from.

Our day-to-day lives *outside* of work can sometimes end up feeling like a never-ending chore. The constant communications, messages that need to be replied to, invitations to say yes or no to, countless decisions to be made, things to buy, house admin to organize. It can feel relentless and adds to the sense of never having time to do the things we *enjoy* in life: read a book, stare out of a window, get lost in thought or be still and quiet and do nothing.

So many of us long to hit pause.

Long to just have everything stop for a moment, so we can take a beat and breathe.

And we forget THAT WE CAN. Quite literally by hitting a button and unplugging from all the devices that keep you connected to the world. I'm talking about a good old digital detox. And not just one where you turn off your devices and then wander lost and bored around your home, but a digital detox where you use the time to really relax, check in and reconnect with yourself and recharge your batteries.

It can be amazingly powerful.

How to digital detox

Step 1: Decide when you're going to have your digital detox and for how long

Choose an amount of time that feels like a treat rather than a punishment. If it feels fun to do a full 24-hour digital detox to kick things off (my preferred way because the results are so instantly phenomenal) then go for it, but if the idea fills you with too much anxiety, start small and do an evening digital detox or just a couple of hours.

Step 2: Think about any practical issues beforehand

If you're doing a full 24-hour or weekend detox, you might want to let your nearest and dearest know how they can get in touch with you in case of an emergency (I've now bought a landline so that I can have a digital detox whenever I want to without having to worry about people being able to contact me in an emergency.)

If you usually use your phone to tell the time, make sure you have a clock or watch you can use instead.

Step 3: Get yourself prepared

Write a list of things you can spend your time doing, for example:

- Read a magazine or a book
- Make something
- Cook
- Draw, paint or collage
- Do some colouring in
- Journal
- Write a short story
- Give yourself a home spa complete with mani-pedi and a facial
- Go for a walk
- Do exercise
- Go to a class
- Have a bath
- Write a friend a letter
- Write yourself a letter
- Create a photo album
- Reorganize your cupboards or drawers
- Stare out of the window
- Reflect and dream
- Meditate
- Play music
- Dance in the kitchen
- Go shopping
- Go to an art gallery
- Meet up with friends
- Get an early night

Write a list of things you can do *with* other people that don't involve a screen:

- Cook
- Dance
- Play cards
- Visit somewhere new
- Walk in nature
- Talk
- Do exercise or play a sport together
- Do a board game or a puzzle
- Plan an adventure
- If you have a partner, you could even have sex! Imagine!

And, of course, you don't have to do anything. In fact, I recommend you allow yourself to get bored, feel the discomfort of it and enjoy it. That is the feeling of your brain not having anything to do for once. Getting bored, being idle, pottering around and doing nothing is so, so important. Because it is how we rest, recharge and reconnect with ourselves. So, don't rush to fill your screen-free time with *doing* things. You also want to spend time just *being*.

Step 4: Switch off and enjoy!

When it's finally time to start the detox, turn those screens off and don't turn them back on until the detox is officially over.

Don't be surprised if it gets a bit emotional.

If you are used to always being connected to the people you love through regular messages, if you entertain yourself with films, TV and social media and if you have realized that you're pretty addicted to your phone, then going on a digital detox can sometimes be quite emotional, particularly if being switched on and busy all the time has been a way for you to avoid being with yourself and your emotions. So, if that happens, be gentle with yourself. Allow yourself to feel the feelings and use the 'Emotional Check-in' exercise (see page 137) to help you process and release any deeper emotions if they come up.

Practising calm

A calm mind is a powerful mind.

When your mind is calm, you are able to access the part of your brain where all the higher thinking, intuition, logic and creativity happen.

The more you practise cultivating a calm mind, the more you will find you will be able to respond to challenges and stressful events from a grounded standpoint and the more you will increase your experiences of contentment, serenity, presence, connection, compassion and peace.

Cultivating a calm state of mind in a frenetic and stressed-out world takes practice and training. And one of the best ways, perhaps *the* best way, to cultivate a calm and present mind, is through the practice of meditation and mindfulness.

When you meditate, you are training the mind to let go of the distractions all around, to focus and come into the present moment, increasing awareness and compassion. Meditation uses breath as a focus, helping you to calm your nervous system and become a passive observer to the thoughts and feelings that pass through your mind.

Mindfulness is the practice of being present and fully engaged in the moment as you go about your day-to-day life.

You can practice mindfulness in whatever you're doing. Meditation trains your brain to focus, observe and be in the present moment and mindfulness is the practice of bringing that into your everyday life.

The practice of meditation and mindfulness is well documented to be life-changing. In a world of non-stop activity and anxious energy, meditation helps you to find that space of calm and serenity within.

A regular meditation practice has actually been proven to change your brain, shrinking the amygdala – the fight-or-flight centre – and thickening the pre-frontal cortex associated with awareness, concentration and decision-making.

It literally helps to turn the volume down on the Shitty Committee and increases your ability to connect with that calmer side of you.

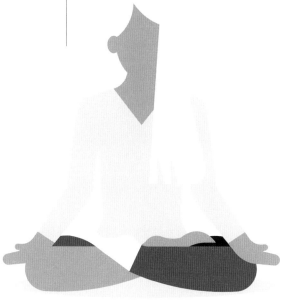

LEARNING TO MEDITATE

There are all sorts of ways you can practise meditation and mindfulness.

My personal favourite is the Headspace app, founded by Andy Puddicombe who trained as a Buddhist monk for ten years before starting up Headspace to bring meditation to the masses.

What I love about Headspace is that it has made meditation something that we can *all* get into, not by dumbing it down, but by showing us easy ways to weave it into our daily lives, no matter how busy those lives get. I love their SOS meditations for those days when you start to feel out of control *and* it has meditations for kids. My son did his first meditation aged four and a half and, to my amazement, he loved it. So, if he can do it, any of us can.

If you've never tried meditation, struggled to get into it or think that it's just not your kind of thing, it is worth giving it another go. I'm going to be totally honest here and say I haven't yet cracked it myself but, in writing this book, I realized that I really do want to get into it. I know it will make such a difference.

My friend Eve is the Director of Meditation at Headspace and the female voice that guides you through many of their meditations. I asked her what to do when, like me, you've struggled to get into meditation and her advice is:

'First of all, don't feel that you are failing if you are not able to make meditation a habit straight away; it is hard starting anything new, especially sitting with the mind, so bringing a sense of kindness to the process is key. The fact that you want to make it part of your life shows that there is intention there, which is also really important!

'Guided meditations are probably best to start with. Start small and build up, even just 5 minutes 2–3 times a week. If you start by saying you are going to meditate every day for 20 minutes you are putting a lot of pressure on yourself and it is much easier to fall off the meditation wagon.

'Each time you do try, think about your intention for why you are wanting to meditate in that moment – it could be something to support you or even those people around you (meditation doesn't just benefit us as individuals it also benefits those around us, too).

'Finally, if you miss a few days, or even a week or so, it is OK! Just come back, start small and pick up from where you left off.'

So set a target for how many times a week you want to meditate to start with, set an intention for WHY you want to meditate and then just get started!

Find your focus, get in flow

When it comes to activity, your mind is at its happiest when it is allowed to fully focus and get in flow. Flow is the state where you become completely absorbed in whatever you're doing to the extent that time seems to fly by or stand still, and you forget about everything else that is going on around you.

Professional athletes, meditators, artists, writers, dancers, musicians and singers often report getting into this state and they call it 'being in the zone'. We can all do it. We are designed to get into this state. But, we can't if we are surrounded by distractions, noise and interruptions, whether from the outside or a chattering Shitty Committee on the inside. We also can't get into that state if we are doing something we don't enjoy – you have to be doing something you love and stimulating for your body, your brain or both.

Flow is the ultimate eustress experience (see page 94), it not only feels *amazing,* but it can help you grow in confidence, skill and ability, and is said to double your productivity and go hand in hand with peak performance. So, it is worth learning how to get into it.

HOW TO GET INTO A FLOW STATE

- You need to be doing something you love
- It needs to feel challenging, but a challenge that you enjoy
- You need to be free of any interruptions or distractions (turn that phone off!)
- You need to be able to focus and concentrate for extended periods of time (meditation can help with this)

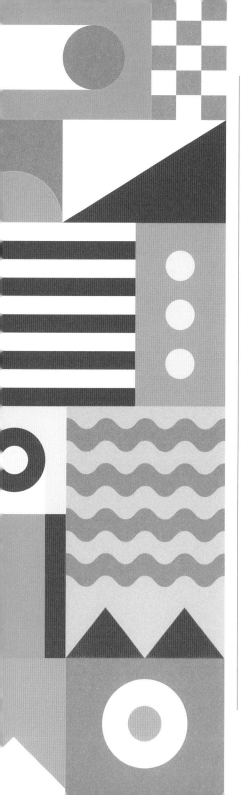

The ultimate goal is for you to have your working day filled with moments of flow. In order for you to get there, your work needs to involve activities and challenges that you love. If it doesn't, then you need to look at how you can bring more of what you love into the work that you do, whether that's making small changes to your current career or changing career altogether – we'll be looking at this in When It's Time for a Bigger Change in Part 3 (see pages 199–211).

What do you need to do right now?

Remind yourself of the key steps to keeping your mind calm, focused and energized (see pages 112 –127) and ask yourself which are you in need of bringing into your life right now?

• What do you need to do to make that happen?

• What is the next step you will take to do that?

Emotional energy

You know the saying 'you can't pour from an empty cup'? Well, emotional energy is the cup.

When you're low on emotional energy, you'll feel like you are running on empty with nothing left to give. Emotional exhaustion happens when you repeatedly put your work, responsibilities or the needs of others before your own and when you try to ignore and suppress your own darker and difficult emotions, such as grief, sadness, anger, resentment, shame, guilt and jealousy.

That doesn't mean, however, that emotional energy is all about being happy, positive and having a smile on your face 24/7. In fact, that is often a sign of someone who is low on emotional energy and trying to pretend that they're fine.

Managing your emotional energy is all about being able to navigate the emotional rollercoaster of life. Of being able to feel your feelings, lean into those darker emotions and, rather than running from them, recognizing that those emotions are here to guide you and show you what you need in order to grow stronger and heal.

You fill your cup by practising self-love, gratitude, connecting with yourself and others in a deep and meaningful way and making sure that you make time in your life for play, fun, adventure, laughter and simple pleasures. They are not nice-to-haves, but essential ingredients without which life will feel dull, monotonous and grey.

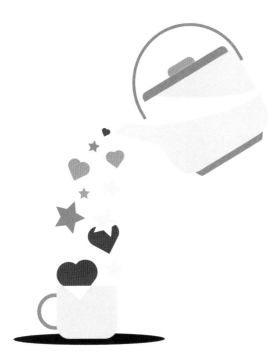

Burnt out from giving

Over-givers are particularly prone to emotional burnout as they tend to give and give and give, not realizing that their energy is limited.

Usually when the cup runs dry for deeply caring, warm and generous people, they can find themselves struggling to feel empathy or compassion for those they care for. Instead they find themselves feeling irritable, resentful and living on a short fuse. And it is heartbreaking when they know they're being like that because that is often the last person in the world they want to be. Then come the feelings of guilt and shame – it's a downward spiral.

Emotional burnout is a big issue among nurses, midwives, doctors, social workers, teachers, therapists, front-line workers and anyone in a caring profession. The relentless demands of the job, inadequate recovery time and neglecting their own needs in order to look after the needs of others means that huge numbers of people in these professions often wind up with compassion fatigue. Their emotional cup has run so dry that they don't even have the capacity to care any more. It's not that they don't want to, it is quite simply that they can't.

This, I believe, happens particularly to over-givers, people in caring professions, parents and carers because of a deep-rooted, crazy, patriarchal notion that those that care for others somehow don't have needs in the same way as other people do. That they are filled up with the very joy of being able to care for and attend to other people's needs.

And it simply is not true.

NO AUTOMATIC REFILLS

We all operate the same way. We all have to manage our energy in the same way.

No one has a magic emotional cup that thrives off neglect and automatically fills itself up every day. We all have a limit to the amount of emotional energy we can give to others. So, no, you can't just give and give and give and not expect to burnout or break down.

If you love to care for people and are there for them, you have to invest the same amount of energy into caring for yourself and being there for yourself. Because when you do, not only will you recover your joy and love for life, but you will also have *more* to give to those around you.

Now, if you're not an over-giver or don't have roles in life where you have to look after the needs of others, it doesn't mean that you don't have to worry about your emotional energy. People who get absorbed in work, keep themselves to themselves, don't invest in their relationships or fail to make time to have fun and enjoy life, will also find their cup empty or stagnant from lack of use.

Emotional energy can be the one I struggle with and resist the most, thinking it's an area I don't need to work on because I'm a naturally enthusiastic person. But, enthusiasm is not a measure of emotional energy. Your ability to make your needs a top priority and speak to yourself with love and encouragement, your willingness to be vulnerable and lean into your emotions and the depth and quality of your relationships is the measure of emotional energy.

HOW TO FILL YOUR CUP

We all have to learn how to keep our cups full and flowing, here's how:

Make time for simple pleasures

Simple pleasures are so, so important. Buying yourself fresh flowers, lying under the shade of a tree on a sunny day, a warm hot chocolate and a piece of cake on a cold winter's afternoon, a hot bath with essential oils, watching your favourite film, snuggling in front of a fire...

These small things have such power to lift our spirits and remind us of the beauty in life.

Start a list of what your simple pleasures are in life – anything that brings joy to the senses – and make sure you treat yourself to them on a regular basis. It will make more of a difference than you might think.

_____

_____

_____

_____

_____

_____

_____

_____

_____

_____

_____

_____

_____

_____

_____

_____

_____

_____

_____

_____

_____

_____

Find the fun

There is nothing that fills up and replenishes your cup quite like the joy and happiness that comes from having fun, playing, being creative, enjoyable challenges and having adventures, and yet so often it is something we reserve only for when we go away on holiday – that is not enough.

We need to bring play, fun, creativity, laughter and adventure into our day-to-day lives. We need to prioritize this and recognize the power it has to light us up from the inside and fill us with energy.

This can be as simple as listening to a podcast that makes you laugh, learning a new fun skill such as calligraphy, or dancing around your kitchen like no-one's watching. If you know you need more joy in your life, write down the things you love doing (or would love to try) that are fun, playful or creative, or the challenges or adventures you'd love to do. And then start making time for them.

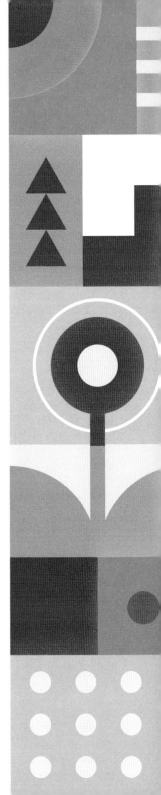

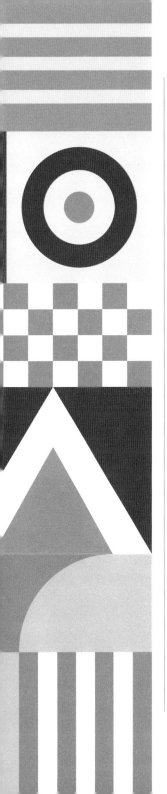

Exercise to get an immediate boost of feel-good hormones

Oh, hello again! Yes, exercise is a great way to fill up your emotional cup as well as energize you physically and mentally. When you exercise, your body releases a cocktail of feel-good hormones that immediately makes you feel happier, more confident, more capable and less anxious. It is an instant mood booster. So, next time you're feeling out of sorts, get that body moving and see how it lifts your spirits.

Practise gratitude

I know practising gratitude is listed in almost every self-help book out there, but just in case you're *not* yet doing it, I thought it was worth mentioning the power of it when it comes to boosting your mood and filling up your cup. Practising gratitude has been proven to increase happiness, empathy and self-esteem, reduce depression, aggression and stress, and strengthen your resilience. It is such a powerful practice that over time it's been found to even change the brain.

There are all sorts of ways you can weave practising gratitude into your day. It can be anything from writing down five things you're grateful for, to going out of your way to say thank you to people, to writing a gratitude letter to someone you really appreciate (whether you send it to them or not).

Make friends with your emotions

Life is a beautiful rollercoaster of emotions and to keep your emotional energy full and flowing, you need to learn how to ride that rollercoaster.

Rather than trying to ignore, hide, suppress or run away from the darker or more difficult emotions, you need to learn to lean in, feel them, own them, accept them and let them guide and show you what it is you need so that you can grow.

The problem is that most of us have been taught to bottle up our feelings, brush them under the carpet and pretend that 'I'm fine' – and it doesn't work.

You can try to pretend those feelings aren't there, but that doesn't make them go away.

When you refuse to *own* your emotions, when you try to pretend that you don't have all the feelings that you have, when you try to appear happy and in control the whole time, your emotions *don't* just disappear.

Quite the opposite.

As American professor Brené Brown once said, 'When you deny your feelings, they double down and grow. And not only that, but they invite shame along to the party.'

And then they tend to wreak havoc in your life. You can find yourself making choices and taking actions that are destructive by nature. When I'm in the grips of anxiety, panic, fear or shame and *I'm pretending I'm not*, I'll pick fights, self-sabotage, procrastinate, blame and turn in on myself. It's not pretty.

So, when you start to feel upset, angry, sad, lonely, ashamed, guilty or any darker, heavier, uncomfortable emotion, you need to take time out and attend to those emotions. Really let yourself feel them without judgement and find out what they are trying to tell you.

Emotional check-in

This is a simple five-step exercise that will help you feel your emotions:

Step 1: Let yourself feel your feelings

The first thing you need to do is to fully accept and embrace how you're feeling by expressing how you feel. Write it out onto a page, talk it out into a voice memo or share how you're feeling with a friend.

A lot of us struggle to articulate how we're feeling or identify how we're feeling. I really struggle with it. If you do too, here are some starting points to help you:

I feel sad that...
I feel angry...
I feel afraid...
I feel worried...
I feel guilty...
I feel embarrassed...
I feel ashamed...
I feel ashamed to admit...
I don't want people to find out...
I wish...
I feel resentful...
I hate...
It makes me upset that...
I feel disappointed that...
I feel irritated by...
I feel fed up that...
I feel jealous of...

Step 2: Understand where your feelings are coming from

- What has happened to make you feel this way?
- What is the story you're telling yourself?
- What expectations do you have of yourself, of others or of life that is making you feel like this?
- What is your Shitty Committee telling you that is making you feel this way?

Step 3: Let it all out

Sometimes, acknowledging how you are actually feeling can bring it all up to the surface and intensify it for a moment. In which case, you might find you need to cry, scream (into a pillow), jump up and down or move your body to feel and release the energy of that emotion.

Shaking is a brilliant way to release energy from the body – it is a Qi Gong exercise that has you shaking your body from your pelvis while your body remains relaxed. (Search the internet for 'Qigong shaking exercise' for a demonstration of how to do it.) It is SO powerful in helping you to regulate stress and emotions. It will shake you down back to the ground if you're feeling agitated or will shake the energy and power back into you if you're feeling deflated. I was taught to use 'shaking' on The Bridge Retreat (a deep-healing retreat). We would literally shake out anger, shame, grief and sadness as it came up. And wow did it work.

Step 4: Let your inner Wise Cheerleader take the mic

- What does your wise, supportive inner self have to say?
- What words of encouragement would you love to hear right now?

You'll be amazed at how your own words can give you the love, support and even wise guidance that you need. Or call a friend if you need to hear some words of love, support and reassurance from someone else.

Step 5: Give yourself what you need

What can you do for yourself right now that will help you?

- Do you need to focus on self-care?
- Do you need to up your levels of self-love?
- Do you need the support of someone who loves you?
- Do you need to get out into nature?
- Can you ask someone for help?
- Can you reassess your goals?
- Can you give yourself some more time?
- Do you need to cancel some plans to give yourself some space?
- Do you need to take a break?
- Do you need to seek some advice?
- Do you need to ask for support?
- Do you need to do the Shitty Committee exercise (see pages 46–7)?
- Do you need to do something that will help calm your nervous system?
- Do you need to do some exercise to boost yourself with feel-good hormones and also boost your confidence?
- Do you need to move or dance?
- Do you simply need to allow yourself to acknowledge your feelings without trying to fix them?

Don't feel you need to move quickly out of the darker, deeper emotions of grief, trauma, sadness and anger. Sometimes you might simply need to allow yourself to acknowledge how you're feeling and why you're feeling that way. Simply make sure you have the support and nourishment you need as you go through it.

Learn to love yourself

Self-love is the ultimate power source when it comes to emotional energy. In fact, it is the ultimate power source when it comes to living a happy and fulfilled life and is a topic that I am fascinated by and passionate about.

So much so that in 2013, Vicki Pavitt and I started Project Love to challenge the modern day narratives around love and to show people that 'when you truly love yourself and become THE source of love in your life, your life will transform from the inside out.'

When you are able to love yourself, life becomes so much easier and more enjoyable. The volume on your Shitty Committee is turned right down and the volume of your inner Wise Cheerleader is turned right up throughout most of your day.

Self-love increases your levels of happiness, contentment, joy, peace, connection, self-esteem, confidence... all the good stuff.

When you love yourself, you believe in yourself, you support yourself, you forgive yourself and you protect yourself. When you love yourself you don't let people treat you like crap and you don't stick around in a job that is burning you out – you make sure that the way you live your life and the work you do makes you come alive and makes you feel good.

Far from being selfish, as people sometimes fear, when you love yourself you have more to give to the world. You naturally want to share the love you have within you. You become *more* giving, generous and loving.

Learning to love yourself isn't easy. I would say it is a work in progress for most people through all of their life.

But, when you start to practise loving yourself, I promise you it will completely change your life.

Here are some of the top tips we share at Project Love to help get you started:

• Journal to connect with your feelings, your thoughts and your inner Wise Cheerleader

• Practise self-acceptance and compassion through meditation

• Get the healing that you need

• Take yourself out on solo dates

• Treat yourself to pamper nights in, just you and yourself

• Keep turning down the volume of your inner Shitty Committee

• Keep turning up the volume on your inner Wise Cheerleader

• Do one simple, loving thing for yourself every day (at Project Love we run a '28 Days of Love' campaign every Valentine's Day to encourage people to flex that self-love muscle by doing one loving thing for themselves every day for 28 days. It is so simple, but so incredibly powerful.

HEAL YOUR HEART

I don't know anyone who has really learned how to love and care for themselves and stepped into their full power without going on their own healing journey.

Many of us are walking around carrying unprocessed pain not only from our own past, but also from that of our parents, grandparents and ancestors. This unexpressed grief, with the related emotions of anger, sadness and fear, can be unwittingly passed down through the generations. It quietly drains away at our emotional energy, holding us back from experiencing deep connection with others and ourselves. Unprocessed grief has also been increasingly linked to a range of medical conditions – from IBS and migraines, heart disease and certain forms of cancer, through to anxiety, depression and addiction. According to Donna Lancaster, co-founder of The Bridge Retreats, it can play a big part in your burnout.

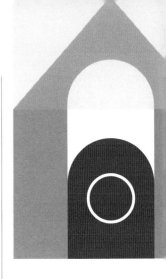

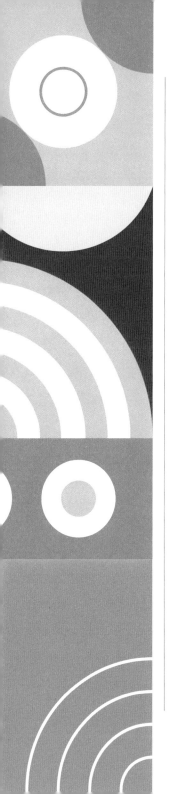

Donna Lancaster is truly the greatest facilitator of healing I have ever come across. She believes that in western society we are often unable to process our losses and the related grief that accompanies them because most of us are not shown how to. She says:

'Many of us grew up within the "stiff upper lip" culture and family system. Instead we are led to believe that only the "good" emotions are allowed and of value. What this leaves us with is individuals walking around carrying so much pain that they have denied or hidden for years, which then, like a poison, turns inward and festers, mutating into conditions like depression and/or gets directed outwards, especially towards those closest to us. Unexplained bursts of anger unfairly heaped on those we love, for example. It is only when we dare to face our pain and grieve our losses, that we can truly begin to heal from them.'

If you often experience feelings of sadness, anger, guilt, shame, anxiety or depression, or you use alcohol, drugs, work, busyness or anything else to try to keep those feelings at bay, then investing in your own healing could be the most important thing you ever do for yourself.

I honestly believe that we all need to make healing a lifelong practice.

Because with every old wound that you heal and every limiting belief you dissolve, you experience more joy, peace and fulfilment in life. And, a greater connection to yourself and others.

FIND THE TOOLS TO HELP PROCESS TRAUMA AND PAIN

If you are a front-line worker or in the armed forces and you see people go through trauma or experience it yourself on the job, then you need to find tools and practices that help you to effectively process that trauma.

You *have* to. That trauma will not disappear, no matter how hard you try to push it down. No one should be sacrificing their mental health and well-being to look after the rest of us. I've spoken to paramedics, midwives, doctors, nurses and social workers as research for this book and it is clear that there is not enough training and support given to most people in caring professions to help them deal with the trauma that they witness on a daily basis.

And while I would love nothing more than to see all front-line workers given powerful and effective trauma training by those that hire them, I don't want any front-line workers waiting a second longer. Talk therapy, somatic therapy, yoga nidra, CBT (cognitive behavioural therapy), EMDR (eye movement desensitization and reprocessing) and TRE (trauma and tension release exercises) are among some of the practices that are said to be particularly good with helping people process trauma – try things out and find what works best for you.

Cultivating good relationships

We all need deep, loving relationships and authentic connections with the people around us to truly thrive in life, not just for our emotional health, but for our physical health.

A Harvard University study of Adult Development that has been going on for eight decades has revealed that those of us with close, supportive relationships live longer, happier, healthier lives than those without. A study of women suffering from breast cancer carried out by the University of California found that those with a strong, supportive circle of friends were four times more likely to make a full recovery. Our friendships literally have the power to help us heal. And they are instrumental in helping us keep our cups full. So, we all need to dedicate time to cultivating deep bonds, nourishing relationships and meaningful interactions in our lives with the people around us.

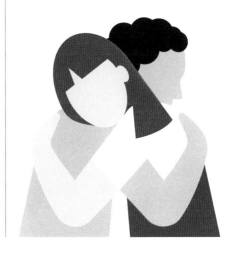

To do that you need to:

- Fill your inner circle with people who show you love and respect

- Find ways to engage in meaningful conversations every day

- Spend *quality* time with the people you love, where they have your full focus (phones off)

- If you manage people, make sure you take time to sit down with them and ask how they are doing and then listen without interrupting

- Reach out and let the people you love know that you're there for them by checking in and asking how they're doing

- Thank the people that you love and who support you for being there for you

- Be vulnerable with the people you love. Take off the mask and the armour and let yourself be seen

- Allow yourself to be helped and supported (don't try to always be the strong one that does all the giving)

- Connect and create community (on or offline) with people who share your sense of purpose

- Find opportunities to be of service, through the work that you do, through volunteering and mentoring or through random acts of kindness

SAY WHAT YOU NEED

Feeling able to ask for your needs to be met is an essential tool when it comes to filling up your cup and protecting your energy on every level, particularly your emotional energy.

Wherever you share space, time, work or household responsibilities with other people, at certain times you're going to have to let those people know what you need and ask for their support in getting that; for example, asking your colleague that you don't get emails or messages about work on the weekend or asking your partner to look after the kids on a Saturday morning so you can have some 'me-time'. If you have never been good at asking for what you need or when you've been brought up to believe that a good and caring person should be accommodating and look after other people's needs, it can sometimes be excruciating when you first have to practise expressing what *you* need.

Deep down we can feel ashamed and guilty about having needs (this is amplified when you're a mother) and that shame can often bubble up as resentment, anger, blame or passive aggression (or just straight-up aggression). Instead of calmly and naturally expressing our needs, we can end up ambushing the other person when they least expect it, already feeling defensive and ready to fight for our needs – and we all know how that conversation goes down.

Your tone, your body language, even the words you use, will immediately leave the other person feeling blamed and attacked. Your underlying message is that you are exhausted and miserable and it is somehow their fault. All they will be focused on is defending themselves and the injustice of your underlying accusation that your unhappiness is their fault and they have somehow been selfish, and then everyone is upset. This guarantees that your needs have not been heard, let alone met.

In order to express your needs and really have them be heard, you need to go into these conversations with your nervous system calmed right down, your inner Shitty Committee out of the room and you need to be willing to be honest with yourself and the other person.

You need to dare to be vulnerable.

And you need to take full responsibility for not looking after your own needs.

Don't be the victim.

It won't help.

The right conversation

Ask the other person when would be a good time to talk – don't just spring it on them. This is an important conversation that requires focus, energy, empathy and attention. If they are busy, distracted, tired, hungry or focused on something else, it's not usually a good time. So, find a time that works for you both to have a chat.

When it comes to having the conversation, if you feel awkward, uncomfortable or emotionally charged, then own it. Express it. It will make sense of your defensive body language, inability to hold their gaze or any other weird, shifty signals you might be giving off. When you're open and vulnerable you open the channels to connection and wholehearted communication.

Say what you need and how you need them to support you in having that need met and you will hopefully find that things flow a whole lot better.

BUILDING HEALTHY BOUNDARIES

As much as you need to learn how to fill your emotional cup, you also need to learn how to protect it.

Remember, you do not have a limitless supply of energy, so you have to create healthy boundaries to protect it and stop yourself from giving it all away to the point where your emotional energy bank is overdrawn and your cup is dried up.

When you have weak boundaries, you'll often feel like your time and energy are not your own. And you'd be right. Without boundaries, or without being able to uphold your boundaries, you can find yourself saying yes a lot because you struggle to ever say *no*. For that reason, you're often the person that friends, family and co-workers turn to when they need a favour. You're also the person that needy or narcissistic people are drawn to because without firm boundaries they can use you as their own personal source of energy.

Now, we all like to help one another, but when you are regularly saying yes to things you simply don't have the energy or time for, and are putting the needs of others before your own needs, day in and day out, then it's a one-way street to burnout.

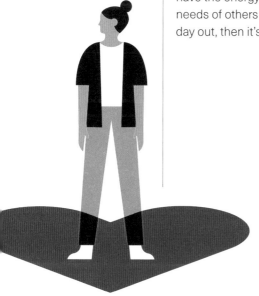

It won't surprise you that over-givers tend to struggle with boundaries more than anyone. It's also something that a lot of women and those who identify as a woman struggle with, regardless of whether they have over-giving tendencies or not. This is because for a long time women have been told that their role is to be accommodating, to say yes even when they want to say no, to look after other people's needs and not have any of their own. This is why setting boundaries can feel so deeply uncomfortable for so many of us, because it involves getting comfortable with saying 'no', speaking your truth, asking that your needs be met and having the courage to take up space in the world. And for many of us that sounds *terrifying*.

If you're an over-giver or a people pleaser (usually one and the same) and your identity is all tied up in being needed, then speaking your truth and saying 'no' feels like social suicide. It's likely that you rely on people's approval to validate yourself, so saying no to someone risks making them unhappy and losing their approval. And your Shitty Committee cannot handle that.

And if you have low self-esteem, low self-worth and are used to playing small and dimming your light, the idea of voicing your needs and limits can feel utterly horrifying. So, I get it, laying boundaries can feel uncomfortable – scary even. It takes courage at first. But, let me tell you, as someone who was once terrible with my own boundaries and had to learn to set them in both my personal and work life, at first it can be a bumpy ride, but it is one of the most powerful things you can learn to do.

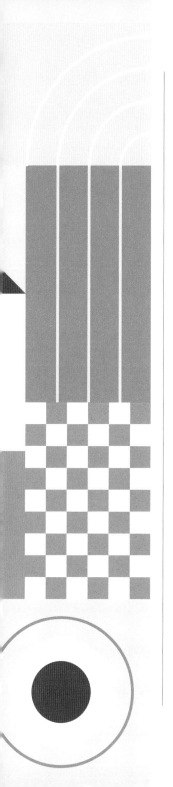

Learning to say no

No matter how uncomfortable it may sound, if you want to stop living life from an empty cup and burning out from over-extending yourself, then you are going to have to start saying 'no'. At first it *will* probably feel hard, you probably *will* find it uncomfortable and people really might *not* like it.

Saying 'no' will go against every people-pleasing bone in your body, but you have to stay strong and do it because if you can't, then you are powerless in being able to protect your own time and energy.

You can say your 'no' lovingly, but don't apologize for it and don't make up excuses – there's no need to lie. You have the right, as does everyone else, to say 'no'.

It's not being mean, it's not selfish, it's simply you being honest about the capacity of your energy and time. For example, if a co-worker asks you to look over a report they've done, but you're already at full capacity, you can say that: 'I'm at full capacity right now.' *If you want*, offer to take a look at it at a later date when you know you'll have more time. Saying 'yes' would have you over-extending yourself and stressing yourself out. For someone else. Why would you say yes to that?

Or say your friend invites you out for dinner on the night you'd already booked to be a night dedicated to rest and relaxation as part of your ongoing commitment to your well-being. You might say something like, 'What a great idea, I'd love to go out for dinner with you, but tonight I can't – how about we do something on... (and suggest another day).'

Now most people will be absolutely fine about you saying 'no', but you will find some people don't like it, particularly if they've been used to always getting a satisfying 'yes' from you to their every request. They might even try to pile on the guilt to get you to change your mind. If they do that, stay resolute. Remember why you are doing this.

When I started practising saying 'no' for the first time, I had a few occasions where people didn't like it. It was hard. But the moment passed, they didn't stay mad forever and, for the first time in my life, I felt like I was able to really protect and look after myself. What I also found was that the people that were at first shocked at me saying 'no' started to practise saying 'no' themselves.

By giving yourself permission to lay down healthy boundaries, you will find you give other people-pleasers in your life permission to lay down healthy boundaries too. And soon everyone's cups will start to fill up again.

What do you need to do right now?

Remind yourself of the key steps to keeping your mind calm, focused and energized (see pages 130–152) and ask yourself which are you in need of bringing into your life right now?

- What do you need to do to make that happen?
- What is the next step you will take to do that?

_____

_____

_____

_____

_____

_____

_____

_____

_____

_____

_____

_____

_____

_____

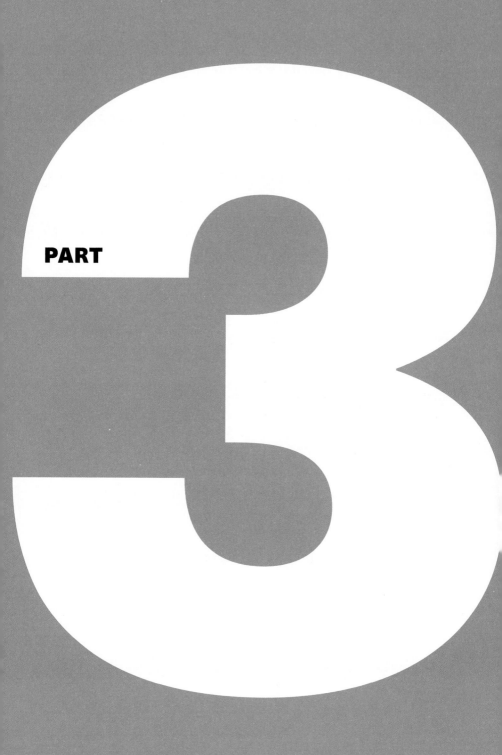

PART

3

DESIGN A LIFE YOU LOVE

Living a life you love does not happen by accident. People who truly thrive in life, who have a career they love, rich and nourishing relationships and enjoy their day-to-day way of living, haven't just fallen into that life.

They have *created* that life for themselves.

They have taken the time to get clarity on what they want and need in their life in order to thrive.

They have had the courage to dream and then the commitment to make those dreams come true.

They have repeatedly taken on their Shitty Committee and their ego, doing the often difficult and challenging work of shining a light on those inner limiting beliefs, fears and ego-driven desires so that they no longer have a hold on them or stop them from living their true potential.

They have dared to create the life that they really want to live, rather than the life they were told they *should* be living.

Dare to design

Creating that life that you love isn't always easy, but, it is oh so worth it. There is nothing more exciting in life than realizing that you really can design the life you want to live.

In fact, as a human being, you were born to do it. You have the magical ability to dream things up and then through intention, belief, action and commitment make those dreams happen. Why would we all be born with this powerful ability if we weren't supposed to use it?

Living your life according to what you think you should be doing or what others have told you that you should be doing won't lead to happiness, fulfilment or even real success– it will lead to a feeling of emptiness, frustration and restlessness. A nagging sense that something is missing, that there must be more to life than this.

For you to live a life that you love, a life that you thrive in, you need to design a life that has you prioritizing the things that are most important to you.

Your day-to-day must have the ingredients you need to thrive woven into it and your career has to have you doing things that make you come alive and nourish your soul.

DARE TO DREAM

When you're feeling burnt out, that kind of dream life can feel like it's impossible and a long way out of reach. But, I promise you, if that is the life you want for yourself then, step by step, you'll get there. Even with just the first few steps you'll start to feel the magic happening. You'll start to feel a shift in energy and your future will start to open to you, suddenly pregnant with possibility as you start to allow yourself to dream and realize that you can change your life.

I have been helping people to create lives and careers they love for the past decade, and the magical results never fail to blow me away.

Watching people go from feeling stuck, miserable, burnt out and lost to feeling energized, alive, back in the driving seat of their life and excited for what lies ahead never fails to leave me feeling moved and humbled at the transformation people are capable of when they put their minds and hearts to it.

Do *not* expect to completely redesign your life in one week. Like any big change in life, you need to give it time and take it step by step. But I promise you the moment you commit to creating the life that *you* want to be living and start taking the steps to creating that life for yourself, you will start to feel the power and magic and realize that you really do have what it takes to create a life you thrive in.

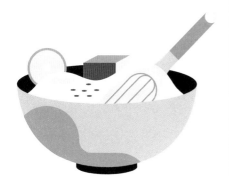

The ingredients you need to thrive

The first step in designing your life is to get clarity on what you want your life to be full of. What ingredients do you need in life in order to thrive?

Using Part 2 of this book to inspire you, start building up your very own bespoke list of ingredients, tools and practices that you feel you need in your life to help you remain energized, calm, grounded and happy as you go about your day (no matter how busy your day gets) – use the examples on the following pages for guidance.

Don't worry if you find yourself repeating some of the same ingredients – this just shows which ones are particularly powerful for you. And, if there is a question that you struggle to answer or don't have an answer for, then don't worry. This helps you to identify areas that you need to spend some time exploring, to discover what works for you.

WORK OUT WHAT INGREDIENTS YOU NEED TO THRIVE

Nourishing yourself

What breakfast meals help you to nourish yourself at the start of the day?

___

What nourishing foods do you enjoy eating at lunchtime?

___

What nourishing snacks help you to keep your energy up between meals?

___

What foods do you enjoy eating in the evening?

___

(See page 68 for inspiration.)

Energizing yourself

What activities help energize your body?

___

Switching off

What activities help you to switch off after work?

___

What activities help you to switch off from work during weekends (or whenever you have time off work)?

___

What activities help you to switch off from work when you're on holiday?

___

(See page 193 for inspiration.)

Resting your mind

What helps you to rest your mind and renew your mental energy when you're on a five-minute break at work?

___

What helps you to rest your mind and renew your mental energy when you're on a 20-minute break at work?

What helps you to rest your mind and renew your mental energy when you're on your lunch break at work?

(See page 112 for inspiration.)

Relaxing

What activities help you to release the stresses of the day?

(See page 70 for inspiration.)

What activities or practices help you to fully relax your body?

(See page 76 for inspiration.)

Good-quality sleep

What conditions do you need for a good night's sleep?

What time do you need to get into bed to get a full 7–8 hours' sleep?

What helps you to wind down and get ready for sleep?

(See page 78 for inspiration.)

Enjoying the simple pleasures in life

What are the simple pleasures you enjoy in life?

Fun, play, creativity and adventure

How do you like to have fun?

How do you like to play (or how did you like to play as a kid)?

What creative activities do you enjoy?

What kind of adventures do you enjoy?

What lifts your spirits?

What do you do when you want to be inspired?

A calm mind

What activities help calm your mind?

What practices help you to cultivate a calm mind?

(See page 122 for inspiration.)

Getting in flow

What activities do you love to do?

What activities do you love to do that can have you completely absorbed for hours?

What environments do you thrive in?

What environments do you enjoy spending time in (it can be specific places or kinds of places)?

What environments do you like to work in?

What environments do you like to relax in?

What environments do you go to when you want to feel inspired?

What environments do you like to be in when you reflect and dream?

What environments do you feel your happiest in?

What environments do you feel most at peace in?

Spending time alone

What do you enjoy doing when you're spending quality time on your own?

Connecting with others

What do you enjoy doing with the people you love?

Who are the kinds of people you feel most comfortable and uplifted by?

How do you meet those kinds of people?

How do you connect with people in your community?

YOUR MOST POPULAR INGREDIENTS

You will probably notice that there are a few activities, practices, people or places that have come up more than once. This is good because it means that these hit a number of sweet spots for you all in one go. For me, it's being out in nature, journalling and exercise.

Which of these ingredients do you want to weave into your life on a daily basis? For example, meditation, exercise, going to bed before 11pm.

_____

_____

Which of these ingredients do you want to weave into your life on a weekly basis? For example, a digital detox evening, spending time in nature, hanging out with friends.

_____

_____

Which of these ingredients do you really want to weave into your life once a month? For example, painting, getting out of town, listening to live music.

_____

_____

Which of these ingredients do you really want to do once a year? For example, a retreat, a holiday to a place you love, a course, a weekend away with friends, a festival.

_____

_____

Now, you should have a juicy list of ingredients to help you feel energized, calm, focused and connected throughout the day.

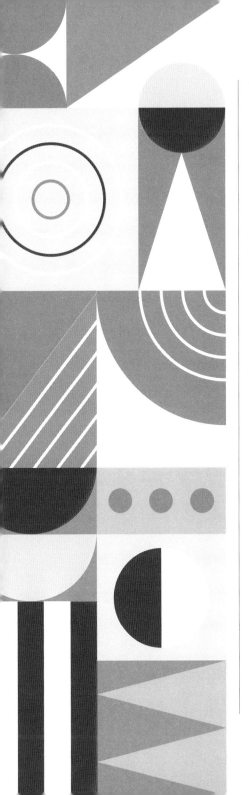

Your life design tools

Now that you have the ingredients you want to weave into your life, it's time to learn the tools that will help you to do it.

TURN YOUR INGREDIENTS INTO NEW HABITS AND RITUALS IN YOUR LIFE

Choose the top two ingredients you want to weave into your life right away. You're going to turn these into habits or rituals that will eventually become a natural part of your daily life.

Getting these habits to stick will take a bit of effort at first, but eventually you'll do them without even thinking.

Creating new habits and rituals that stick

For each of the ingredients you want to turn into a daily habit or ritual, write down:

1. **Exactly what are you going to do?** For example... have a digital detox evening.

_____

_____

_____

2. **When are you going to do it?** For example... Tuesday and Wednesday evenings.

_____

_____

3. **How are you going to remind yourself to do it?** For example... I will schedule it into my calendar and put an alarm on my phone to remind me to switch it off.

_____

_____

4. **What are you going to do to make it as easy as possible for you to stick to this new habit as it takes hold in your life?** For example... I will write a list of things I'm looking forward to doing during my digital detox.

_____

_____

5. **How will you feel doing it?** For example... I'll feel rested, relieved and free!

_____

_____

_____

Start small

If you've chosen to do something that is going to take no more than 5 minutes and feels really easy to do, then you might want to commit to doing it 5 to 6 days a week.

If it's something that requires a good amount of time and/or effort to do, such as 10 minutes of meditation or 30 minutes of exercise, then start small. You might want to commit to doing it just 1 to 3 times a week.

We want you to succeed at this, so make it easy for yourself!

Experiment to find the best time in the day

It might take a while to find the right time in the day or week to weave in your new habit or ritual. For example, if you want to get into a meditation practice you might find it's great to do in the morning to set you up in the day, at lunchtime to help you calm your nervous system and renew your energy or in the evening to help you relax before bed. Try it out at different times and see what works best.

MAKE SPACE IN YOUR LIFE

Our daily lives are made up of habits that we don't even think about. We often think we don't have a spare minute in our lives, only to find that when we switch off our screens we suddenly have a surprising amount of time on our hands.

Take a look at what existing habits you could switch out for a new practice you'd like to weave into your life. For example, if you usually wake up in the morning and reach for your phone to check the news, messages or social media, you could replace that morning habit with journalling, meditation, getting out in the garden, stretching, reading an inspiring book or poems. Whatever it is you choose, replace your phone on your bedside table with something that reminds you, or helps you, to do that new activity instead.

If you want to weave something into your life that takes 30 minutes or more of your time, look at how you can move things around to make space for it. Remember that with time, you never find it – you have to create it. By shifting your schedule around a little bit, you can create space in your life to do something that could totally change your day... and your life.

Get creative and experiment to find out what works best for you. Ask yourself:

- Can you get up half an hour earlier to do it?
- Can you leave the house half an hour earlier to do it?
- Can you do it on your way home?
- Can you do it in the evening after work?
- Can you make time for it on the weekends?

REMIND YOURSELF

If there is an activity you want to do at a specific time in the day, then put an alarm on your phone or, if you want to keep things analogue, put a post-it note somewhere that you'll see it at the right time.

In the book, *Atomic Habits*, James Clear recommends 'habit stacking' where you can attach your new ritual or habit to an already existing habit or routine. For example, if you would like to introduce a 30-second yogic coffee breathing exercise into your morning to wake up your body and mind, you could do it as you boil the water for your morning cup of tea.

Or if you already take a walk every morning (walking the dog, walking your kid to school or walking to the station), you could turn that walk into a gratitude walk where you mentally write a gratitude list each morning.

I have a friend who has a 40-minute commute to work that she turns into her meditation time. She finds her seat on the bus, plugs in her headphones, closes her eyes and by the time she gets to her destination, she has calmed her mind and is focused ready to take on the day.

MAKE IT EASY

Early morning exercise is a habit that a lot of people want to get into, but one that a lot of people fail at because when that alarm goes off at 6.30am, the last thing most of us feel like doing is jumping out of bed to go for a run.

The key is to make it as easy as possible.

Lay out your workout gear the night before. If you're doing yoga at home, lay out the yoga mat the night before too, so it is ready and waiting for you.

Book yourself into morning exercise classes to give you that extra commitment. Agree to do exercise with a friend (it's much harder to let our friends down than ourselves). Or, as one of my friends does, head off to work in your exercise gear (with your work clothes in a bag), having not had a shower. It will force you to head into the gym if only to shower before work and, once you're in there, well, you might as well hit the gym.

IT CAN TAKE EFFORT AT FIRST

Don't be surprised if, even though you are designing ingredients into your life that you really want to do, you find yourself resisting them at first. Old habits die hard, and with every new habit you are weaving into your life, an old habit is being pushed aside.

As behavioural change specialist Shahroo Izadi says in her brilliant book, *The Kindness Method: Changing Habits for Good*, 'Whether we like it or not, the habits we've developed to distract ourselves from our uncomfortable thoughts and feelings have, at some point, been effective and useful – otherwise we wouldn't have clung onto them for so long.'

So, go gently, keep at it, and if you fall off the wagon you can always get back on.

GETTING BACK ON TRACK

You might get off to a great start weaving these new ingredients into your life but, at some point, the chances are you'll fall off track. More than once.

Life will throw you challenges, you'll feel like you don't have the time, you'll feel like it's not working. It will feel too hard, you'll feel too tired and your Shitty Committee will tell you it's not possible and will encourage you to give up on the whole thing. Your natural response will be to drop all your new good habits, throw this book in a drawer and reach for your old coping mechanisms. When that happens, I want you to remember this: falling off course and wanting to give up is an inevitable part of this journey.

You will fall. You will return to your old habits. You will want to give up.

And that's OK.

Do not use it as a stick to beat yourself with. You haven't failed. You have simply fallen off course. And now you can choose to pick yourself back up and use the following five-step process to get you back on track.

Five-step process to getting back on track

Step 1: Forgive yourself
Remind yourself why you wanted to start this journey to begin with.

Step 2: Get curious
What happened to throw you off course, and what can you do the next time that happens? What is your Shitty Committee saying about it?

Step 3: Recommit
Remind yourself why you are doing this. Why is it so important? And let your inner Wise Cheerleader give you a pep talk or a message of encouragement.

Step 4: Take action
Show your commitment to getting back on course by doing something that helps to give you a burst of feel-good energy.

Step 5: Celebrate!

Your canvas for life

When it comes to designing your life, your calendar is your canvas.

Plenty of us use calendars in our day-to-day lives to keep on top of things at work and in our home life. But the magic happens when you start to use it to design the life you want to live.

If you don't already have a calendar for your personal life, it's time to get one. Whether a digital or paper calendar, it needs to have hourly slots so that you can clearly design your day, dedicating specific times to the things you want to do.

I use a digital calendar so that I have it on my laptop and phone, and so I can share it with my partner. It also makes it easy for me to colour code things: pink for work projects; dark green for coaching sessions; light green for well-being activities; yellow for fun stuff; blue for appointments and other life admin; orange for anything related to my son.

By colour coding my different activities I can quickly see how my week is looking and whether I have enough fun and well-being activities in there. It quite literally becomes my canvas for designing my life.

MAKE IT HAPPEN

However you choose to use your calendar, the key is to develop a strong relationship with it.

You need to know that whatever goes into your calendar *will happen*. So you need to check in with your calendar the night before to remind you what you have to do the following day.

Use the reminder alarm to help stick to your commitments to yourself and others, and always check your calendar before saying 'yes' to someone.

When you know that whatever goes into your calendar has to happen, you will have the power to design the life you want to live. You'll have the confidence to know that whatever you put your mind to, it will happen. Rather than allowing other people's needs and plans to fill up your life, you'll start filling it up with your needs and plans first. And there is nothing more powerful than that.

Using a calendar can seem like such a trivial thing. A time-management tool, that's all. But, when you learn how to use it and you develop a real commitment to doing what is on your calendar, you will discover that it is so much more than that. It is a tool that can help you to reclaim your time and live the life that you really want to live.

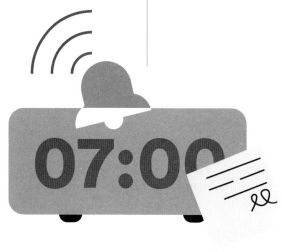

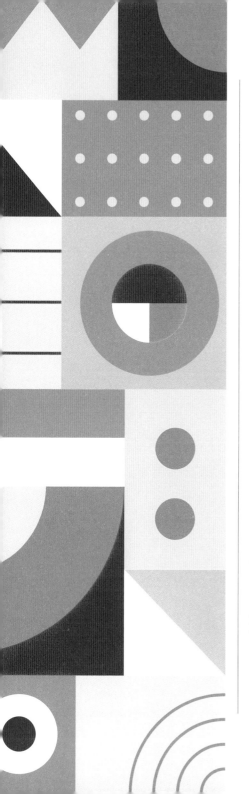

SOMEONE TO CHEER YOU ON

Daring to make your happiness and well-being a top priority in life, taking on your Shitty Committee in the process and bringing about long-lasting change in your life are all difficult things to do. They take commitment, time and energy and it can make a big difference when you have people by your side, wanting you to succeed, cheering you on, holding you to account *and encouraging you back on track when you fall off.*

So who might that person (or people) be for you? How can you ask them to support you?

Maybe they're working on projects and dreams in their own life, in which case perhaps you could support one another and meet up once a fortnight, in person or online, and share how you're getting on, what you've been up to, any ways that you are struggling and what you're going to focus on over the following fortnight.

But, even if you don't have someone to do this with, let those that want to support you know what you're up to and share with them regularly how you're getting on. Celebrate each step forward and let them cheer you on.

Design your working day

In order to break free from the burnout cycle and really start to thrive, we have to find a new way of working. We have to be the pioneers, the rebels, the revolutionaries who choose to take regular breaks throughout the day, who turn their phone off in the evening, who won't check emails before going to bed and who switch off fully from work on the weekends and allow ourselves to enjoy life. And you know what, as a result, not only will you be the most energized and happiest person at work, you'll also be the most productive and effective.

So let's take a look at how you can design your working day so that you can give yourself the conditions you need to thrive.

Good morning!

How you start your day sets the tone for the rest of it. This is also precious time for yourself.

You already dedicate enough of your day to work, so when you're at home, *be at home*. Make that time for you.

If you tend to start your day by reaching for your phone or laptop and check emails, social media or work messages, then it's time to stop and reclaim your mornings for yourself.

Let's take a look at what you can do to start your day the right way.

ENERGIZE YOURSELF

When it comes to getting energized in the morning, there are so many small things that can make a big difference.

Here are some simple things for you to try out:

1. **Drink a big glass of water when you get up**

   We wake up dehydrated, and dehydration plays a big part in fatigue. A big glass of water first thing is an immediate energizer.

2. **A cold blast in the shower**

   At the end of your normal shower, give yourself a blast of cold water for 30 seconds (or more if you can bear it). Not only will it give you an immediate energy and mood boost, it will boost your immune system as well, and leave you feeling alert and invigorated.

3. **Yogic coffee (30 second breathing exercise)**

   If you haven't tried it, give it a go (see page 75). It is amazingly energizing. I first tried it when I was regularly waking up feeling exhausted and it was like magic and way more powerful than a real coffee. It gives you a huge burst of energy while simultaneously calming your nervous system.

Mornings are a great time to exercise, if you are able to. That might be 30 minutes of walking, stretching, HIIT, dancing round your kitchen or energetic housework. Getting your body moving, your heart pumping and your brain flooded with oxygen, along with the cocktail of feel-good hormones that are released during and after exercise, is a great way to kickstart your day.

For a lot of people I know, bringing exercise into their morning routine has been life changing. It is worth trying it out to see if it works for you – if it does, it might be worth getting up that little bit earlier to fit it in. However, always be mindful of your energy and listen to your body. Some days a HIIT workout might be exactly what you need, and other days a gentle 20-minute yoga routine might be more suitable. Always allow flexibility in what exercise you do.

GROUND YOURSELF

It's so important to start your day feeling grounded. What helps you to feel grounded?

- Journalling
- Meditation
- Yoga moves
- Exercise
- Dance
- Breathing exercise
- Setting an intention for the day
- Connecting with nature (watering your indoor plants, getting out in your garden if you have one, or walking in nature)
- Reading positive affirmations
- A few minutes of stillness
- Writing what you're grateful for
- A message to you from your inner Wise Cheerleader
- Listening to music

If you're not sure what does it for you, experiment and try things out. Discover what helps you to start the day feeling grounded and make it part of your morning every day.

Your day at work

Now the game is on. It's at work where all the burning out happens and where the biggest transformation has to happen for most of us.

This is where you need to become a master of managing your energy otherwise it is going to be drained left, right and centre by the people around you, intense work sessions, challenges and pressing deadlines. This is where people are going to push your buttons, and your Shitty Committee will find reasons to come charging in and throw you into a panic or have you doubting your abilities.

Let's look at the tools you can use to design your day so that you can manage and protect your energy and consequently be at your happiest and most productive.

As you read through each section, choose two tools that you think will make the most difference and start designing them into your day immediately.

SCHEDULE BREAKS

Taking regular breaks is one of THE most important things you can do to keep your energy topped up throughout the day. No more slogging your way through the day as if you were a machine – that's a recipe for burnout. It's time to get in sync with your natural ultradian rhythm (see page 114 to remind you of why this is so important): schedule 20-minute breaks into your day every 90 minutes or so and you'll immediately feel the difference. You'll be more focused, more energized, smarter and more productive. It's an instant game changer. If you have a day that is often filled with meetings, book in a mid-morning, lunch and mid-afternoon break for 20 minutes (more for lunch if you want) and schedule meetings around that. If your day is free of meetings, set a timer every 90 minutes to remind you to take a break.

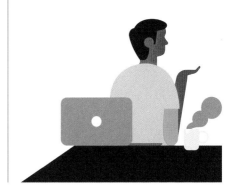

Now, obviously some days won't go to plan – a client may call you out of the blue just as you are about to take a break or you get called into a meeting – so sometimes your work session might stretch for 2 hours and sometimes you'll only be able to grab a 5-minute break. But, something is better than nothing, and, over time, you'll find that those breaks will become more and more important to you as you realize what a difference they make. As that happens, you'll find you get better at making them a top priority.

And on the days that you feel like you just don't have the time to take a break, remind yourself that you will do better work, make better decisions, be smarter, more alert, calmer and more compassionate if you do.

What if you can't take a break?

If you're currently in a situation where you have very little control over your working day once it gets started and even the idea of being able to take a break when you want is laughable, then see what you can do for now. Be creative. If you're rolling your eyes thinking 'she has no idea – I could never do that', meet me in the next section, When It's Time for a Bigger Change on pages 199–211, because we need to talk about making some longer-term changes to how you work and where you work.

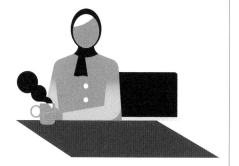

USE BREAKS TO RENEW YOUR ENERGY

It's not just taking time to step away from your work that is important, but what you do in that break.

Whether you take a full 20-minute break, or manage just 5 minutes, make sure you do something that really helps to renew your energy, calm your nervous system and get you back to feeling the way you want to feel. If you're an extrovert and you've been working on your own, then you might want to have a chat with someone (extroverts get their energy from being with other people). If you're an introvert who's been in meetings, then you might want to go and spend some time alone (introverts get their energy from being alone).

If you're doing something that uses up a lot of physical energy, use your break to relax your body and stimulate your mind. If you've been glued to your screen using a lot of mental energy, do something that gets your body moving and stretching and helps your brain to switch off from work (see page 192–3).

If your work involves being there for other people, use your breaks to fill up your emotional cup (see page 133), and if you've been doing intense work that has got your adrenaline pumping and into a state of distress or even the healthy eustress zone, use the break to calm your nervous system (see page 96).

Find spaces to do some deep-focused work

This is absolutely essential.

Unless you have work that never requires your full focus or attention, you *need* to have a space that you can go to where you can do deep-focused work and not be interrupted.

Open-plan offices (or any place of work that is full of people, noise and interruptions) can be a hotbed for stress and burnout, and also one of the worst places to get any serious work done. The interruptions and distractions are *endless* and crazy making. From colleagues asking you questions, to people chatting around you, phones ringing, music playing, the photocopier whirring, the coffee machine bubbling... the list goes on.

According to a study by Steelcase, people in open-plan offices are interrupted or distracted on average every 3 minutes and, according to a study on productivity carried out by the University of California, when you're doing deep-focused work it can take about 23 minutes to get back on track after an interruption.

Ideally, where you work would offer quiet 'do not interrupt me' rooms. If it doesn't, see what you can do to create that for yourself with what you have to hand.

- Are there meeting rooms that you could use?
- Could you work some days or mornings from home and do your deep-focused work there?
- Is there a café where you can escape to?
- If you work from home and also struggle to get peace and quiet due to lack of space and a noisy household, could you transform your bedroom, a spare room or the kids' room into a pop-up work space for the day?

And if all else fails, a pair of noise-cancelling headphones and a big sign that says DO NOT DISTURB on your door or your desk should hopefully keep most people away.

Move, stretch and breeeeeathe

Remember the importance of moving, stretching and breathing throughout the day to help keep your energy topped up and your mind alert (see page 70). It is absolutely key to helping you remain energized. Remember, you can habit-stack (see page 168), for example stretch and take three slow deep breaths whenever you're making a cup of tea, standing at the photocopier or going for a bathroom break. Or, put a reminder alarm on your phone to do it every hour.

Keep fuelled

If you don't have nourishing food that you love to eat and that is easy to get your hands on when you're at work, invest a bit of time, using the tips on pages 66–9, in setting yourself up so that you have the lunch and snacks you need and want to fuel you through the day.

Keep hydrated

It is so easy to forget to drink water during the day and dehydration is a huge cause of fatigue and brain fog. So, if you know you're not very good at drinking water during the day, invest in a nice water bottle or jug and fill it up at every break. It is one of the easiest ways to boost your daily energy.

Turn off *all* of your notifications

If you haven't already turned off every notification on your digital devices, then do it now. If you need a reminder of why it's so important, see page 104. And, while you're at it, make sure you don't have any notifications popping up on your computer screen or, if you have one, your smartwatch. Get them out of your life!

Do one thing at a time (no more multi-tasking)

If you need a reminder as to why multi-tasking kills your productivity, concentration, creativity, emotional intelligence and lowers your IQ, then see page 110.

If you're struggling to focus, or find yourself procrastinating, use the Pomodoro Method (see page 111).

SOS tools

If you're having a difficult or stressful time at work, use the following tools to help:

Feeling stressed?

Take a time out and help yourself shift from distress to eustress using the Stress SOS tools on pages 96–7.

Feeling out of sorts?

When you feel fed up, unmotivated, angry or upset or just out of sorts, take a time-out and help yourself to move through those feelings. Give yourself what you need using the Emotions Check-in on page 137.

Feeling overwhelmed?

Grab a piece of paper and get everything out of your head and on to the page.

Feeling tired?

Step away from your screen and take a break – move, stretch, get some fresh air, do the yogic coffee breathing exercise (see page 75) or have a nap. Don't accept tiredness, lethargy and fatigue as the norm. Recognize it as a sign that you need to do something to boost your energy. All it takes is a couple of minutes!

Feeling like you can't do it?

Any time you start doubting yourself, feeling a loss of confidence in your abilities or notice that you're suddenly looking at the situation or yourself negatively, it is a sign that your Shitty Committee is in town. And the moment it is, you need to put down your tools, step away from what you're doing and get to work tuning into what your Shitty Committee is saying and turning its volume right down (see page 46). And make sure you also take a moment to turn the volume UP on your inner Wise Cheerleader (see page 54) so that you walk away feeling empowered and back on track.

Yes, you *can* do this!

Protecting your energy at work

One of the things that can make working such a hotbed for stress is the fact that you have other people to deal with. Other people who are also getting stressed, feeling under pressure and with their own Shitty Committee on their backs.
Not to mention the narcissists and egomaniacs.

Now, I don't have many tips on how to handle the toxic bosses, other than *leave them* (more about that on page 204), but there are some things you can do to handle the time thieves, crappy bosses and difficult colleagues who can drain your energy and your time like nothing else.

TIME THIEVERY

One of the biggest problems I hear from people working in teams is how often their time is wasted by people bringing them into meetings, or email threads, that they really don't need to be involved in, as well as the late-night texts invading their home time that could easily be left to the following day.

Now, if that time thief is a demanding narcissistic boss, there probably isn't a great deal you can do to change their bad practices, but if they are peers or the people you manage, here are some things you can try:

Talk to them
If you can, talk to the time thief about laying down some boundaries around communications, for example no texting after working hours or on weekends or asking you first before booking things into your calendar, and so on. And if they keep doing it, keep reminding them until it sinks in. You might even inspire them to get better at laying their own boundaries around work.

Ask them to be specific

Time thieves rarely realize they are doing it, so when a time thief asks you to meet for a catch up, a phone call, or join you in a meeting and you fear it's going to be a time waster, ask them to clarify exactly what they want to talk about or why they need you to be at that meeting.

Let them know what you have on

If you have a time thief in your life who always needs you to help them out, the next time they do it, instead of saying 'yes', try to let them know that you're at full capacity right now and ask that you postpone for the following week. Not having you immediately to hand all the time while also realizing how busy you are will hopefully make that time thief think twice next time.

Delay your response

Some people get hooked on rapid-fire emailing and texting about anything and everything. I think I've been bad about this myself when I've been on the brink of burnout.

The best way to deal with this kind of time thief is to not get whipped up into their frenzy, and to delay your response. If they don't get the dopamine hit from you, they'll move on and find someone else to do it with.

Ask them if it can wait until you're back at work

When your time thief gets into the habit of texting you in the evening after work or at the weekend, you need to get into the habit of asking them if it can wait until you're back at work. Simple as that. Gently bring them back to what time it is and explain that they are asking you to engage in work out of hours. And, from now on, explain this to them every time they text you out of office hours. If they get irritated and start hounding you, then at that point you need to talk to them.

A lot of us have got into bad practices in the workplace. You might even be realizing that you're a bit of a time thief yourself. Don't give yourself a hard time if you are. What we all need to do is start undoing the bad habits that many of us have fallen into and bring in healthy boundaries that protect everyone's time and energy.

HOW TO HANDLE DIFFICULT COLLEAGUES

Whether they are highly competitive, passive aggressive or moody, managing difficult colleagues can be a huge drain on your energy. Here are some things you can try in order to handle them:

- **Get those boundaries laid down**

  See page 184 on how to set healthy boundaries to protect your energy from energy vampires and mood hoovers.

- **Take a time-out when they trigger you**

  Use the tools on pages 96 and 183 to help you handle your emotions and stress levels when they trigger you.

- **Practise compassion for them *and* you**

  We're all just wounded children underneath it all. I know that might make you roll your eyes, *but it's true*. Practise compassion for both of you.

- **If you can, talk to them**

  Find out what might be going on for them and let them know how you're feeling. See page 184 for a refresher on how to have those tricky conversations without blame and getting people's defences up.

- **Talk to someone else about it**

  If you don't feel you can talk to a difficult colleague, talk to someone neutral and supportive about their behaviour – they might be able to offer a different perspective on what is going on and how you can manage it.

- **Don't be afraid to ask for help if it gets bad**

  Never be afraid to talk to your boss or HR for guidance and support if you have a difficult conversation to manage.

Dealing with inequality and discrimination at work

We live in an unfair and unequal world and it plays itself out heavily in the workplace. Sexism, systemic racism, transphobia, lack of accessibility, ageism, homophobia, sizeism, classism... all the isms and phobias can show up in the workplace and it's scary how much they do.

When you're on the receiving end of discrimination, including the subtle, socially normalized microaggressions, it is painful, it is rage-inducing, it is heart-breaking, it is psychologically distressing and it most definitely contributes to burnout, along with PTSD, mental-health issues and other illnesses.

If you work in a company and you are not cis, white, male, straight, able-bodied, university educated, middle class and child free, then the chances are you're going to experience some sort of discrimination at some point, simply for being who you are.

Is this fair? Hell no. Obviously not.

Should we fight to change it? Of course, and I believe we all need to be working together, each using the privilege that we have, to bring about change and create a fair and just world for all. But, are things going to change overnight or even in our lifetime? Highly unlikely. So, we have to find ways to rise up and thrive anyway.

This is *not* an easy one to navigate, but here are some things that may be helpful:

- Join communities and groups, on or offline, where you can hang out with people in the same boat, share your experiences, ask advice, seek inspiration and help one another rise up. There is something so powerful about knowing that you're not alone and banding together to empower one another.

- Find allies at work – talk about what you're experiencing at work with a trusted colleague – let them know how they can be allies and an advocate for you.

- Get a mentor who is seasoned at navigating the world in the same way as you and who can help and support you as you find your way through similar challenges, while guiding you in your career advancement.

- Read books, articles and watch documentaries about people who have been through similar challenges to you and risen up, to keep you feeling empowered and inspired.

- Know your rights. There are laws in place to stop discrimination, and if you have been treated unfairly or experienced discrimination at work you could have a legal case.

- Advocate for others and be an ally yourself, recognizing and using the privilege you do have to fight and make your workplace inclusive for people who don't hold the same privileges as you. We all need to fight for one another.

DEALING WITH RACIAL MICROAGGRESSIONS AT WORK

Racial microaggressions in the workplace are often a common, sometimes daily occurrence.

'Can I touch your hair?'

'Ooh I'm almost as dark as you now with my tan.'

'Where are you from originally?'

'I don't see colour.'

Being invited to a meeting you know you wouldn't normally be invited to so that your company can appear to be 'diverse'.

Nova Reid, an anti-racism educator, describes racial microaggressions as, 'A form of everyday discrimination, every-day comments, behaviour and "othering" that communicates to a person in an ethnic minority identity, that they are somehow misplaced and that they don't belong.'

She explains, 'Racial microaggressions are the ways everyday racism sneaks up in the workplace, as well as in relationships, WhatsApp chat groups and even around the family dinner table and they can have a detrimental impact on well-being.

'In isolation they seem harmless. That's what makes them so difficult to tackle, because when you're on the receiving end of them it can lead to you feeling paranoid or even like you are going "crazy". This can impact everything from self-esteem, confidence and sense of belonging, to your ability to thrive and your overall life satisfaction. Research on racial trauma also shows regular exposure to racial stress, such as microaggressions can show up in the body – specifically Black bodies – as post-traumatic stress disorder.'

While it is most definitely for White people to take ownership of the racism that runs through the fabric of our societies and transform it, while we wait for that to happen, here are a few tips from Nova on how you can handle racial microaggressions in the workplace should they happen to you:

'Firstly, ascertain if you are safe: There is a risk, when calling out everyday racism, that you will receive further abuse or be gaslit. So, consider, do you, personally, have the capacity to engage (it's not your job to call out every microaggression) and is this interaction worth the risk?

If safe, decide if you want to address it in the moment or retrospectively, and try the following:

1. '*What you did there...*' (repeat what they did or said).

2. '*That hurt me' / made me feel* xxx' / '*That was offensive*.'

3. '*I wanted to let you know because I care about our relationship / my community and it causes harm*.'

If you're not feeling safe or don't have the capacity, (because, let's face it, it's exhausting and difficult), this is where allies or support networks are important. Don't keep it to yourself – you are not being paranoid – go there to have your experience heard, seen and validated and if they can advocate on your behalf, even better.

Increase your self-care as a priority.

'Regular exposure to racial microaggressions have such a detrimental impact on our well-being and they aren't going anywhere anytime soon, so do everything you can to boost your emotional and physical well-being, without apology. Say no, delegate, get creative, sing, dance, paint, exercise, try something new, go out in nature, do whatever nourishes your soul.'

If you're White and want to help make your place of work a safe space for Black and Brown people, then the best thing you can do is to learn, shine a light on your own inner racism (we have it within us whether we like it or not) and bring the conversation to the workplace. Nova has called me out on my own inner racism before, and not only did our friendship survive (and no, it was not comfortable), but it deepened.

As Nova says, 'Microaggressions are a form of suppressed prejudice, they are going to happen and it's often kind, caring, well-meaning people who commit them. Consciously making a decision to take responsibility and address them is key to helping reduce harm.'

Dealing with patriarchy at work

Anyone who says gender inequality is a thing of the past is a cis, White, straight man who has managed to spend their life living in a bubble of male privilege, completely oblivious to the daily struggle many women have to put up with in the workplace and sometimes even at home.

It's the gaslighting that does it for me. Not just the ignorance that this happens, but the denial that it does.

Over the years, I have watched one woman after another smack into the glass ceiling as they rise up in seniority in companies, until they come face to face with the white male ruling elite that dominates over 75 per cent of the directors/boardrooms and realize the reality and enormity of the inequality in which we are still deeply entrenched.

And those who become mothers can find that they now have two discrimination battles to fight as they find themselves suddenly invisible, written off, no longer a viable option for promotion and, in some cases, edged out of their role altogether.

If it were just my many clients over the past decade that I'd seen go through this, you could argue that I was just seeing the unfortunate cases, the exceptions, due to the nature of my work. But, I have seen a huge number of my female friends go through it, too. It is happening everywhere, all the time, and it is one of the biggest factors that has my female clients wanting to change career altogether to start up on their own. Because they are tired of it all. The discrimination, the glass ceiling, the pay gap, the inequality, the sexist comments, the being talked over, being looked down upon, the mansplaining and the gaslighting.

After years of having to put up with it, to find that in the end the white men still rise to the top just for being white and male, and they grow tired of it all. Tired of the fight. And they leave.

I'm not going to lie, I've seen many of those women who leave discover that they can thrive so much better when they no longer have to work in a world that wasn't designed for them to win in it anyway. But, I appreciate that not everyone wants to quit or can quit. In which case, follow the points in this chapter so that you protect and support yourself as much as possible.

The system is broken, but don't let it break *you*.

At the end of the work day

With the lines between work and home so blurred these days it is essential that we all deliberately and mindfully put clear boundaries back in place, transitioning out of work mode and into home mode, so that the home once again becomes a sanctuary free from work.

Create some simple rituals to help you switch off from work so that you can fully engage in your home life. For example:

- Check your diary to remind yourself what you have on the following day, so that you can feel mentally prepared
- Decide on the three things that you're going to focus on the following day and write them down
- Tidy up your workspace and leave it ready so you can get started straightaway when you get in the next morning
- If you work from home, tidy all work-related tools away and close all the tabs on your laptop in case you want to use it later when you're in HOME mode
- If you have a journey to and from work, use it. Just like you can use it to get into the right mood and mindset in the morning, use your journey home to start the unwinding and switching-off process as you head home: listen to your favourite music, call a friend, take a walk through a park, do exercise
- As always, experiment with a few different things and see what activities help you step through your front door feeling refreshed, fully disengaged from work and ready to enjoy being at home

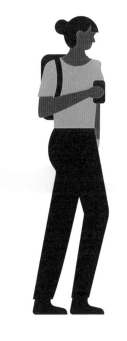

RELEASING THE DAY'S STRESSES

If you are still feeling the stresses of the day, do something to help you calm your nervous system.

Here are a few things for you to try:

• **Shake** – if you're feeling stressed or overwhelmed, try shaking it out. It's incredibly effective and can take just a few minutes for you to feel the effects.

• **Exercise** – this a great way to help you release the stresses of the day and renew your energy, help you to get out of your head and into your body, and flood your body with feel-good hormones.

• **Get out in nature** – nature is the perfect soother. Get your shoes off and your feet on the earth, put your back against a tree and feel it support you, look out at moving water, gaze up at the sky, while taking slow deep breaths.

• **Breathe in some calming essential oils** – certain smells have an incredibly calming effect: lavender, bergamot orange, chamomile, lemon. Have some calming essential oils on your desk, in your bag or in your bathroom and use them to give yourself an instant hit of calm when you need it.

• **Hug** – oxytocin, known as the cuddle hormone, has been found to be released along with cortisol when we get stressed. Which means that our bodies are literally telling us to go and get a hug when we're stressed out. And for some people it can be an instant soother. You can get a hug from a loved one or from yourself. Yes, I promise it works. Wrap your arms tight around yourself, take a slow deep breath in and start gently patting yourself soothingly. It works a treat for me. I never want to let go! Having an orgasm is also a great way to release oxytocin that will help you feel calm and mellow again. Just saying!

• **Talk it out** – sometimes simply talking about how you're feeling and acknowledging to someone that you're feeling stressed and panicked can help to calm you down.

• **Laugh** – you can't laugh and feel stressed at the same time. So, if you're feeling stressed out, find something that makes you laugh and you'll notice the stress lifting straight away.

• **Meditate or do a visualization designed to help you release stress** – these are powerful stress busters. Headspace have some brilliant guided meditations to help you release stress including a three-minute stress buster that you can do any time you need it.

• **Have a hot bath** – after a stressful day, a hot bath or hot shower can really help your body and mind to relax and help your stresses to melt away as more of that delicious oxytocin is released into the body as your body warms up.

MAKE TIME FOR YOU

When you get home from work there may well be another to-do list waiting for you: dinner to prepare; clothes to wash; maybe children to wash; house admin to do blah, blah, blah. I get it. I have to do it all, too. But, among all this you also need to dedicate time to doing things for *you*: things that help you to renew your physical, mental and emotional energy. They don't have to be big – you can start small – 10 minutes of reading before bed; a relaxing bath; catching up with a friend; playing a game; making something with your hands; dancing around your kitchen; cooking your favourite meal.

These things might *seem* small, but if you dedicate just 10 minutes a day to doing something purely for your own enjoyment, happiness and well-being, those 10 minutes of me-time can end up making a big difference.

IF YOU DO NEED TO DO SOME WORK

There may well be times when you simply do need to work in the evenings (but make sure they are few and far between). If that is the case, still make sure that you dedicate part of the evening to being deliberately work-free and dedicated to doing something enjoyable for yourself such as something that helps you to reconnect and lift your spirits.

WHAT IF YOU WORK NIGHTS?

If you work night shifts, get home in the early hours of the morning and usually crash straight into bed, create some rituals that don't take too long and some that even start on the way home to help you to get into home-relaxation-this-is-my-sanctuary mode.

Then, create space the next day to have that down time where you stay away from the emails and work and focus on giving your body, mind and soul what it needs to fully recharge and revive.

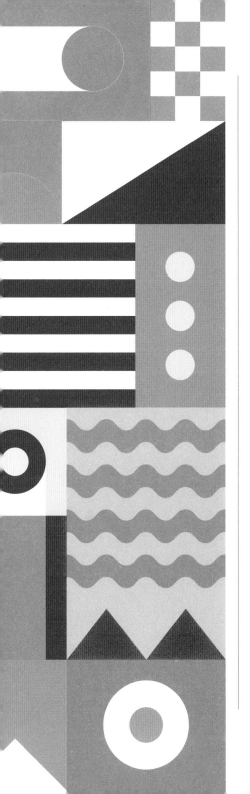

Give it time

And there you have it, a new design to your working day. One that is literally designed to help you thrive.

As I've said before, go slow when you're making long-lasting changes to your life. Don't expect to do it all overnight. Choose the part of this working day that you felt would make the biggest difference to you right now and start there.

Then once that's woven into your life and you're doing it with ease, choose another part of your day to work on. And, step by step, you'll get there.

When it's time for a bigger change

As you make changes to your day-to-day life and feel your energy and your strength beginning to come back, you may start to see that there are some areas of your life that need some serious change in order for you to thrive.

You might realize that you need to leave your company, close your business, change career, leave your relationship, move country...

PREPARE YOURSELF

Whatever the change and whatever the reason for doing it, be prepared that it is always going to feel scary. And even when the change is something you feel excited about, like a dream you want to go after, the chances are your Shitty Committee will *not* like it.

Because making a change always involves stepping out of your comfort zone and taking a leap of faith into the unknown... which is your Shitty Committee's worst nightmare. So expect it to fight against you, fill you with doubt and fear, and try to convince you that it's a terrible idea and it is much better to stick with what you know, even if it is making you miserable. At least it is safe.

And that is why creating a life that is designed for you to thrive in always takes courage. Because no one ever falls into living a life they love by accident. Never. Not even the most privileged among us. It always takes courage, it always takes daring to follow your own path in life and it always takes stepping out of your comfort zone and into the unknown.

Whatever change you want to make, there are a few key steps that you need to take:

Be clear on what you want

At first, all you might know for sure is that you want to quit your job, quit the city or move to another country, but knowing what you want to get away from, won't help you move forward. You need to take time to reflect and get clear on what you *do* want.

Don't hold back when you're dreaming of what you want your future to look like. Too often we let our Shitty Committee have us play small and not dare to dream of what it is we really want, so instead we create our Plan B life, without even giving Plan A a chance. If there is one thing I have learned over the years, it's that if you can dream it and believe in it, you *can* make it happen. So, don't hold back – allow yourself to dream up the life you really want to be living and go after that.

Get inspired

Find people who have been in a similar situation to you and made the kind of change you made. It will encourage you that it is possible and will be great ammo to turn down the volume on your Shitty Committee.

Explore and experiment

Don't go thinking that you have to have everything figured out and a foolproof plan before you get started on your journey. *It doesn't happen that way*. You're going to have to commit to making the change and start taking action long before you really have a clue of what you're doing. It's by exploring, experimenting, talking to people and trying things out that you will find your way, step by step.

Get guidance, support and help

When you are going through a big change in life, it is scary and there will be challenges along the way. So, don't try to do it all on your own. Get the guidance, help, support and advice you need to help you along on your journey, whether that's emotional support from friends, a coach to help you make the change or advice and tips from someone who has already made a similar change to the one you want to make.

Remember your own inner Wise Cheerleader

While your Shitty Committee will hate you making any kind of change in your life, your inner Wise Cheerleader will *love* it and will want to be cheering you on and celebrating your every step forward. So don't forget to tune in regularly to your inner Wise Cheerleader to enjoy the kind of love, support and encouragement you'd be giving a friend if they were in the same position as you.

Break things down

Big change can feel daunting and scary because of the enormity of it, so you need to break it down into manageable steps and focus only on the next step ahead of you. Step by step you'll get there.

Common challenges to expect if you decide to change career

If you're wanting to leave a career that comes with a certain amount of status, then be warned – your ego may not want to let it go. Because the chances are it will have come to rely on that status to feel important and validated in the world. 'Without that status what will you be?', your Shitty Committee will wail in horror.

Well, let me tell you – without that status you will finally be free. At first it may be terrifying if you don't know who you are without it, but once you start creating that inner GPS and anchor yourself to what is really important to you, outside status will lose its power as you start to discover the real power that comes from knowing who you are and what you are here on this earth to do.

It can also be painfully hard to wave goodbye to a career or a business that you went into because you were so deeply motivated to help people. Being a nurse, doctor, midwife, social worker, paramedic or any role where you care for people in their most vulnerable moments is often something, when you go into it, you never imagine you will leave. You go into it because you have a deep, driving desire to help people and then spend many years of hard work, as well as money, training to do that job. And so, leaving it behind can feel like utter betrayal or failure. Often both.

If you're in that situation right now, whatever your career might be, I want you to know that it is not, no matter how much it might feel like it right now, a failure. Failure would be to continue in a career that had you having to abandon yourself every day, that had you having to ignore your body, heart and soul in order to do the work that you do. And, if anything, it is you that has been failed – by a system, by a world that is not designed for you to thrive. The chances are you were led to believe that things would be different. But as discussed, nowhere highlights and intensifies the inequalities, injustices and toxic masculinity in our society quite like the modern-day workplace, whatever your work is.

As Tamu Thomas, a trauma-informed somatic and holistic life coach, says,

'The way that we live, the way that we're conditioned, the patriarchy, capitalist, white supremacy. Those systems are all designed to keep the masses knackered so that the chosen few at the top can be successful and can gain from our labour.

'So, if we want to thrive in life, we have to have the courage to *choose* to thrive in life.

And sometimes that means doing things differently and walking away from the systems that keep us exhausted.'

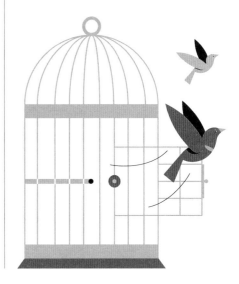

IF YOUR WORKPLACE IS TOXIC... *YOU NEED TO LEAVE IT*

Toxic work cultures and toxic bosses are everywhere.

I never stop hearing about racism, sexism, unlawful discrimination, bullying and narcissism in the workplace.

No industry is immune. I've seen it happen in every industry, not just the corporate world. I've seen it happen in big-name charities, creative agencies, music labels, magazines, fashion houses, the UN, hospitals, start-ups, universities, government, schools... everywhere. The trendiest, most popular, most sought-after places to work can often be the most toxic.

I've lost count of the out-of-court settlements and NDAs I've seen friends and clients sign so that well-known companies don't get exposed for having an issue with in-house bullying, racism, sexism and discrimination. It is happening everywhere and it is being silenced in a big way.

And if it's happening or has happened to you and you're still in that toxic environment, then I really only see one option for you.

You need to get out.

Working for a person or a company that makes you feel worthless, undervalued, second-rate or treated like a machine and not a human, will eat away at a person's self-esteem, confidence and sense of self-worth until you are left totally and utterly broken. Toxic bosses and toxic work cultures are psychologically damaging.

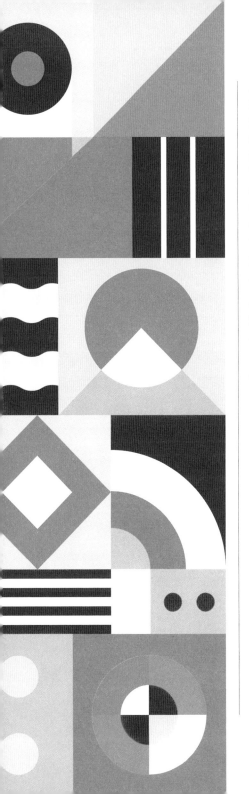

Just as in any psychologically abusive relationship, you will start to think that you are the problem. You're not. You need to get out. I don't mean march in tomorrow and quit. So don't panic. You might need to build up your confidence and your strength first, but what I know for sure is that you can't stay working for a company or boss that pushes you so hard and breaks you down so badly that you burnout.

You are never going to thrive there. All the tools in the world won't help you to do that.

You wouldn't plant a flower in toxic soil and expect it to thrive. So why in the world would you expect the same of yourself?

For you to really get to thrive and be happy in life, you need to be standing as far away from the toxic people and cultures as you can. Leave them to themselves. Screw them anyway, they do not deserve you.

There are other jobs out there and other companies and bosses who believe in treating their employees with respect and care, who work to empower their teams and who make the happiness and well-being of their employees a top priority. So go and find those people and get a job with them.

DON'T PUT MONEY BEFORE YOUR WELL-BEING

If you feel stuck where you are because money is an issue, then I assure you that there is always a way to make the money that you need to thrive in life that doesn't come at the cost of your well-being. I have been helping people change career for over a decade, and in all that time I have not once seen someone unable to change career, or at the very least change jobs, so that they could earn a living and not be made mentally or physically unwell in the process.

And don't go telling yourself that you have to make a choice between happiness and money. That is a limiting belief that a lot of our Shitty Committees feed us: the idea that either you do work that is consuming and hard and brings little in the way of joy or fulfilment, but you get paid well so you can have the home, the car, the holidays. Or, you do work you love, but you live on a tight budget and can't afford the home, the car or the holidays.

Having both simply isn't an option.

NOT TRUE. Of course, you can have both.

But, only if you allow yourself to believe that it's possible. And that brings us back to the rules of the Shitty Committee. If you don't challenge the limiting beliefs it's feeding you, you'll continue to think that they are the truth. So, if your Shitty Committee says you can either love what you do and thrive or make good money, but not both, then you'll often make the following choices to keep living within the limitations of that belief:

- You'll say yes to the job you don't really want because it is good money.

- You'll say yes to doing work you love for very little money or for free.

- You won't even bother to apply for the job that looks great and offers good money because it will seem too good to be true.

- Even when you are presented with the opportunity to do something you enjoy that pays you good money, your inner saboteur will play up, making you take the wrong train so you end up late to the interview, making you ill just as the job is about to begin or filling you with so much self-doubt that you are in a permanent state of stress that you kick into overdrive, your burn-out archetype fires up and, before you know it, the dream job has turned into yet another job that pays good money but makes you burnout. Never underestimate the power of your Shitty Committee to sabotage those great opportunities for you so that it can prove itself right.

As soon as you are clear on the change you want to make, go back and revisit the Shitty Committee exercise on page 46, and get out all the limiting beliefs your SC has around the change you want to make and why it says it isn't possible. Don't let it hold you back.

WHAT IF YOU CAN'T QUIT YOUR JOB STRAIGHTAWAY?

Sometimes you will want to stick it out in a job that is not allowing you to thrive for a bit longer. Sometimes now just isn't the right time to be quitting and finding something new. Sometimes it takes a while for you to build up the strength and the courage. If that is the case, make sure you have a clear plan of when you will be handing in your notice. Even if it is next year. Create a timeline and put that stake in the ground so that you can see the light at the end of the tunnel. Then, do everything you can to look after yourself as best you can in the meantime. Use the tools in this book, make use of the time you do have, no matter how little, to really rest, relax, recover and do things that bring you joy.

If you're going to stick it out in a job that makes you miserable and exhausted for a little longer then do it strategically and mindfully – don't be a martyr to it.

Find the help you need: get a coach, join an online community that is all about well-being, get some friends to be your support crew. Do everything you can to support yourself in looking after your emotional, physical and mental energy while you stick it out in an environment that was not designed with your well-being or happiness in mind.

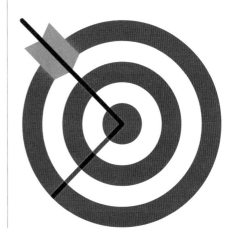

A STOP-GAP JOB AS AN INTERIM SOLUTION

If staying in your current job a day longer feels too much, then get what I call a stop-gap job. A job that lets you get away from the one that is making you ill to help you pay the bills, but that also leaves you with enough energy and time to focus on figuring out the longer-term plan. Find a job that you find easy to do, possibly dropping down a position or going part-time to achieve this.

I've known people to do this and then find that the stop-gap job turned out to be a great option for them, freeing them up to follow passions they didn't have time for previously, and they ended up settling into it for the long term and being happy.

SOMETIMES YOU JUST NEED TO REPACKAGE WHAT YOU DO IN A DIFFERENT WAY

Making a change doesn't always mean changing your career. Sometimes how you do your work, where you do it or who you do it for needs to change, but what you do can remain the same, if perhaps in a different package.

Sam, one of my earliest clients, was a burnt-out marketing director working all hours at a marketing agency. He ended up changing jobs to work in-house for a big brand where he was free of the constant demands from clients (now that he was the client) and he got to leave every day at 5pm and focus on a photography business he had decided to start on the side after having rediscovered his love of photography.

Maeve was a burnt-out and bored doctor who thought her days in medicine were over when she came to see me. After some digging, we discovered that it wasn't medicine she was tired of, but the lack of adventure and physical challenge in her life. She ended up working as a medic in the Antarctic for a year. It gave her the adventure she was craving and rekindled her love of medicine.

Sameera was an overworked and burnt-out lawyer in a London law firm. She quit her job and started to work as a freelance lawyer and found that she suddenly had far more freedom, time and the work-life balance she longed for.

Other people have taken parts of their career that they loved and repackaged them to do what they love in a way that they love.

Penelope was Global Strategy Director at an international magazine group and was possibly the most burnt-out person I have ever met in the most toxic environment I have ever heard of.

She took her talent and love of nurturing teams, in particular helping women find their direction and their voice, and her experience navigating complex work situations in a white, male dominated world and pivoted to start up her own coaching business 'My So-Called Career', helping women take ownership of their careers.

Her business was up and running in no time, and she was booked up with a waiting list within her first year in business.

Alice had been working as a PA and Administrator for 10 years for small charities and media companies, but she was tired and burnt out from working in an office. She wanted adventure, more creativity in what she did and she wanted to help people that were making a difference in the world. She took her experience as a PA and set up a Virtual Assistant business, Virtual Alice, and had her first paying client in under a week. She started learning how to create websites so that one day she could add that to her offering and now that she had an online business, she was finally able to make her dream come true of moving to Madrid.

And Tamu, whose wise words you read a moment ago, quit her career in social work after a massive burnout that almost had her needing a bone-marrow transplant, and today uses that experience and training in Somatic Coaching to coach women (including me) how to thrive in a world that is not designed for them to truly thrive in.

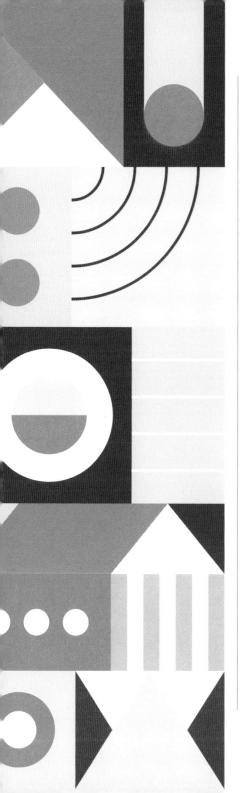

You might think right now that this kind of change isn't possible for you. You might find it hard to imagine – impossible even. But let me tell you something, every one of these people once felt the same. Almost every person I talk to when they first come to me says the same thing at the start: 'Maybe I'm the one person you won't be able to help. Maybe I'll just never find the right career for me.'

To this day I've not met a person who hasn't found work they enjoy doing. As Penelope says, 'Your work should make you feel good. If it doesn't, then it's not the right work for you.'

Does it mean that it's always easy?

No.

Does it mean no day should ever be a struggle?

Of course not.

But if every day is hard and if every day is a struggle, then that is not the right work for you.

You have the power to change. So change it.

Life
beyond
burnout

When your body burns out, it knows what it's doing. It's asking you to stop, to slow down, to take a step back and look at your life and see that the way you are living and working is not working for you. It's not good enough for you.

Yes, the world we live in is a challenging one and, more often than not, an unfair one. But, you were born to thrive. You have the right to thrive. And you can thrive.

Breaking free from the urgent fast-paced way of living that so many of us have got sucked into, isn't an overnight job and it isn't always easy. As Brené Brown says, 'It takes courage to say yes to rest and play in a culture where exhaustion is seen as a status symbol.'

You can be sure that from time to time you will fall off track, life will start to move at a rushed and urgent pace again and you'll find your over-giver, over-thinker, over-doer or over-achiever back in the driving seat.

Remember the tell-tale signs that signal you are slipping into your burn-out archetype? When you notice that familiar feeling of kicking into overdrive and suddenly your self-care habits start falling by the wayside, use the tools in this book to help you slow things back down, reconnect to your body and remember what you need to do to keep yourself feeling energized, calm and grounded.

I promise you, if you commit to learning what it is you need in order to thrive in life and you dedicate yourself to making sure that you have those ingredients woven into every day, then, step by step, you will not only leave those burnt-out days behind you, but you will find you have more energy, more compassion, more peace and more joy in your life than ever before.

And it's when you are filled up with energy that you'll start to be able to live the life and do the work that you are really here to do.

So let's do it.

Let's reclaim our energy, reclaim our lives.

And thrive.

Resources

Let's keep this journey going...

I hope that by now you are starting to feel calmer, more energized, happier and more alive than you have done in a long time. If you keep following the exercises and practices in this book it will happen. And, I hope too that you've started to realize that you deserve to be living a life in which you can thrive – if you're not, then things need to change and I love nothing more than helping people to bring about positive change in their lives. So, rather than this being the end of our journey together, let this be just the beginning.

USE THIS SPACE TO REMIND YOU OF YOUR ESSENTIAL TOOL KIT FOR THRIVING IN LIFE

What I commit to doing daily to help myself feel energized, calm and grounded:

_____

_____

_____

_____

_____

_____

What I commit to doing at the end of the day, every day, to help my body and mind rest, relax and find peace:

_____

_____

_____

_____

_____

MY SOS TOOL KIT

What helps me when I'm feeling overwhelmed:

_____

_____

_____

_____

_____

_____

What helps me when I'm feeling anxious:

_____

_____

_____

_____

_____

_____

_____

What helps me when my Shitty Committee is in town, filling me with doubt, fear and shame:

_____

_____

_____

_____

_____

_____

_____

What I need to remember to do when I feel stress kicking in:

_____

_____

_____

_____

_____

_____

_____

MY DAILY INSPIRATION:

My values:

_____

_____

_____

_____

_____

_____

_____

_____

_____

_____

_____

_____

My purpose:

_____

_____

_____

_____

_____

_____

_____

_____

_____

_____

What my inner Wise Cheerleader wants me to always remember:

ONLINE RESOURCES

www.theburntoutbook.com

Here you'll find bonus resources that accompany this book, plus a guide on how to use this book with friends.

www.selinabarker.com

Head over here to find out all about what I'm up to, my latest products and courses, how to connect with me and how you can work with me.

www.selinabarker.com/themondaycrew

Join The Monday Crew (it's free) to get my weekly mini-podcast dedicated to helping you design a life you love, one Monday at a time!

Instagram @selinathecoach

Follow me on Instagram where you'll find me talking regularly about how to dare to do things differently and design your life so that you can thrive in a fast-paced world.

www.loveprojectlove.com

Tune into 6 years of Project Love podcast episodes where Vicki Pavitt and I explore what it takes to create a life, career and relationship that you love.

brenebrown.com

This is the website for Brené Brown, Research Professor at the University of Houston, containing information, blogs and podcasts that discuss studies on courage, vulnerability, shame and empathy.

www.novareid.com

If you're a White person wanting to find out how to make your workplace a safe space for Black and Brown people, visit Nova's website for her amazing anti-racism training.

FURTHER READING

To keep the inspiration and practical guidance flowing, here are some books to help inspire you.

Allen, David, *Getting Things Done: The Art of Stress-free Productivity*, Penguin Books, 2001 [p.65]

Adegoke, Yomi and Uviebinené, Elizabeth, *Slay In Your Lane: The Black Girl Bible*, Forth Estate, 2018

Brown, Brene, *Dare to Lead: Brace Work, Tough Conversations. Whole Hearts*, Vermilion, 2018

Cantwell, Marianne, *Be A Free Range Human: Escape the 9–5, Create a Life You Love and Still Pay the Bills*, Kogan Page, 2019

Chatterjee, Rangan, *The 4 Pillar Plan: How to Relax, Eat, Move and Sleep Your Way to a Longer, Healthier Life*, Penguin Life, 2017

Gannon, Emma *Sabotage: How to Silence Your Inner Critic and Get Out of Your Own Way* Hodder & Stoughton, 2020

Hendricks, Gay, *The Big Leap: Conquer Your Hidden Fear and Take Life to the Next Level*, HarperOne, 2010

Huffington, Arianna, *Thrive: The Third Metric to Redefining Success and Creating a Happier Life*, WH Allen, 2015

Izadi, Shahroo, *The Kindness Method: Changing Habits for Good*, Bluebird, 2018 [p.116]

Northrup, Kate, *Do Less: A Revolutionary Approach to Time and Energy Management for Busy Moms*, Hay House, 2019

Portas, Mary, *Work Like a Woman: a Manifesto for Change*, Black Swan, 2019

Reading, Suzy, *The Self-Care Revolution: Smart habits & simple practices to allow you to flourish*, Aster, 2017

Sarpong, June, *Diversify: Six degrees of separation, because the world is separate enough*, Harper Collins, 2017

Schwartz, Tony and Loehr, Jim, *The Power of Full Engagement: Managing Energy, Not Time, Is the Key to High Performance and Personal Renewal*, Simon & Schuster, 2005

Wax, Ruby, *A Mindfulness Guide to the Frazzled*, Penguin Life, 2016

PODCASTS

'Unlocking Us' by Brené Brown

https://brenebrown.com/podcast/brene-on-comparative-suffering-the-50-50-myth-and-settling-the-ball/ (accessed 1 September 2020)

'Project Love Podcast' by Selina Barker, & Vicki Pavitt
https://loveprojectlove.com/podcast

'Ctrl, Alt, Delete' by Emma Gannon
https://play.acast.com/s/ctrlaltdelete

'Conversations with Nova Reid'
https://novareid.com/podcast/conversations-with-nova-reid-new-podcast-series/

'The Calmer You Podcast' by Chloe Brotheridge
https://calmer-you.com/podcast

'Wellpreneur' by Amanda Cook
https://wellpreneur.com

INDEX

AUTHOR'S ACKNOWLEDGEMENTS

Writing this book truly changed my life. I am honestly a calmer, more grounded, more energized person today thanks to the journey this book has taken me on, and so I owe a huge thank you to every person who has played a part on that journey. Not only did you help me to write a book that I'm truly proud of, but you helped to change my life for the better.

Thank you to all of you who took the time to write to me and talk about your experience of burnout; you were my inspiration throughout.

Thank you to the Celebration Sisters – you are the reason this book exists.

To Dr Tilean, Donna Lancaster, Tamu Thomas, Nova Reid, Molly Manners, Marianne Cantwell, Penelope Jones, Imogen Felton, Julia Nightingale and Lauren Davey – your insights and wisdom were invaluable in shaping this book.

Thanks to my wonderful business wife, Vicki Pavitt, who helped me shape the idea for the book in the early days and enthusiastically allowed me to try out every exercise on her.

Thanks to Tony Schwartz and Jim Loehr whose ground-breaking work around energy management and book *The Power of Full Engagement* had a huge influence on me.

To my agent, Valeria Huerta, for believing in me and helping to make my dream of writing a book come true.

To Kate Adams at Aster for being brilliant and helping me to shape the book into what it is today, and to the team at Octopus for being a joy to work with.

Thank you to my Dad for showing me that burnout can be the best thing that ever happens to you and a catalyst to go after your dreams, and to my Mum for being so committed to my well-being during all the years when I wasn't. I got there in the end.

And finally, the biggest thanks to Fonz, without whom I could never have written this book. Taking on all that you did so that I had the headspace, time and energy to write a book was a huge act of love that I will forever be grateful for.